O P M L
OXFORD PAIN MANAGEMENT LIBRARY

Opioids in Cancer Pain

O P M L

OXFORD PAIN MANAGEMENT LIBRARY

Opioids in Cancer Pain

Edited by

Prof. Karen Forbes

Consultant and Macmillan Professorial Teaching
Fellow, Department of Palliative Medicine,
Bristol Haematology and Oncology Centre,
Horfield Road, Bristol, UK

OXFORD
UNIVERSITY PRESS

OXFORD
UNIVERSITY PRESS

Great Clarendon Street, Oxford OX2 6DP

Oxford University Press is a department of the University of Oxford.
It furthers the University's objective of excellence in research, scholarship,
and education by publishing worldwide in

Oxford New York

Auckland Cape Town Dar es Salaam Hong Kong Karachi
Kuala Lumpur Madrid Melbourne Mexico City Nairobi
New Delhi Shanghai Taipei Toronto

With offices in

Argentina Austria Brazil Chile Czech Republic France Greece
Guatemala Hungary Italy Japan Poland Portugal Singapore
South Korea Switzerland Thailand Turkey Ukraine Vietnam

Oxford is a registered trade mark of Oxford University Press
in the UK and in certain other countries

Published in the United States
by Oxford University Press Inc., New York

© Oxford University Press, 2007

The moral rights of the author have been asserted
Database right Oxford University Press (maker)

First published 2007

British Library Cataloguing in Publication Data

Data available

Library of Congress Cataloging in Publication Data

Data available

Typeset by Newgen Imaging Systems (P) Ltd. Chennai, India
Printed in Italy
on acid-free paper by
L.E.G.O. S.p.A., Lavis (TN)

ISBN 978–0–19–921880–6

10 9 8 7 6 5 4 3 2 1

Contents

Contributors

Naeem Ahmed
Pain Fellow, St Mary's Hospital,
London, UK

Ganesan Baranidharan
Consultant in Pain Management,
Leeds Teaching Hospitals,
Leeds, UK

Augusto Caraceni
Medical Director of the Virgilio
Floriani Hospice, Palliative
Care Unit, National Cancer
Institute, Milan, Italy

Polly Edmonds
Consultant in Palliative Medicine,
King's College Hospital NHS
Foundation Trust,
London, UK

Marie T. Fallon
St Columba's Hospice Chair of
Palliative Medicine, University of
Edinburgh, Edinburgh Cancer
Research Centre (CRUK),
Western General Hospital
Edinburgh, UK

Chris Farnham
Hospice Consultant, St John's
Hospice, Hospital of St John
and St Elizabeth, London, UK

Christina Faull
Consultant in Palliative Medicine,
LOROS Leicestershire and
Rutland Hospice,
Leicestershire, UK

Luke Feathers
Consultant in Palliative
Medicine, Leicestershire
and Rutland Hospice
and University Hospitals
of Leicester,
Leicestershire, UK

Karen Forbes
Consultant and Macmillan
Professorial Teaching
Fellow in Palliative Medicine,
Bristol Haematology and
Oncology Centre,
Bristol, UK

Stefan Grond
Stellv. Direktor,
Universitatsklink fur
Anasthesiologie und
Operative Intensivmedizin,
Martin-Luther-Universitat,
Halle-Wittenburg,
Germany

Peter Hoskin
Professor of Clinical
Oncology, University College
London and Consultant
Clinical Oncologist, Mount
Vernon Cancer Centre,
Northwood, UK

Jeremy R. Johnson
Medical Director,
Severn Hospice,
Shrewsbury, UK

Matthew Makin
Consultant in Palliative
Medicine and Programme
Lead for Pain,
The Marie Curie Palliative
Care Institute Liverpool and
the Dept. of Palliative
Care Medicine Wrexham
Maelor Hospital, UK

Sandra McConnell
Specialist Registrar in Palliative
Medicine, Western General
Hospital, Edinburgh, UK

Felicity E. Murtagh
Research Training Fellow,
Dept. of Palliative Care, Policy
and Rehabilitation,
Weston Education Centre,
Kings College London, UK

Colette Reid
Locum Consultant in Palliative
Medicine, Gloucester Royal
Infirmary, Gloucester, UK

Eija Kalso
Associate Professor, Dept. of
Anaesthesia and Intensive
Care Medicine, Helsinki
University Hospital, Finland

Karen H. Simpson
Consultant in Pain Management
And Senior Clinical Lecturer,
Leeds Teaching Hospitals,
Leeds, UK

Catherine E. Urch
Honorary Senior Lecturer
UCL and Imperial College
Consultant in Palliative
Medicine, Dept. of Palliative
Care, St Mary's and
Royal Brompton Hospitals,
Paddington, UK

**Giovambattista
Zeppetella**
Medical Director,
St Clare Hospice,
Hastingwood, Essex, UK

Preface

Cancer is increasingly prevalent as our population ages. A significant proportion of patients with cancer will suffer from pain, due to their cancer or diagnostic or therapeutic interventions. The study and management of pain due to cancer has developed enormously over the last three decades, exemplified by the publication of the World Health Organization method for cancer pain relief in 1986, now commonly known as the World Health Organization analgesic ladder. Studies have demonstrated that, using this method, the majority of patients' pain due to cancer can be controlled, however we know that in everyday clinical practice patients with cancer continue to suffer pain and to have their pain inadequately managed. There are many complex reasons for this, but they include professionals' lack of knowledge and ill-founded beliefs and attitudes about the use of morphine and other strong opioids.

In this Oxford Pain Management Library book on Opioids in Cancer Pain we have drawn together the skills of many clinicians routinely using opioids to successfully manage difficult pain in patients with pain due to cancer. We hope this handbook will be a useful tool in aiding colleagues in primary care and the medical and surgical specialties to assess and manage the patient with cancer pain. The book is divided into five parts; a first section on 'Pain in patients with cancer' deals briefly with the aetiology and prevalence of cancer pain and general principles of pain management. The second section on 'The treatment of cancer pain' looks at the range of treatments for cancer, and the relative role of opioids alongside anticancer therapy. This is followed by a chapter on the history and development of the World Health Organization analgesic ladder. The third section discusses the principles of using opioids for cancer pain and dealing with adverse effects. The final two sections consider the commonly used oral opioids in turn and then alternative routes of opioid administration and opioids in special circumstances. The book aims to be evidence based and relevant to clinical practice.

I am grateful to all of the contributors for sharing their clinical experience and expertise. I hope that readers will find the book useful and that it will enable you to approach the patient with pain due to cancer with greater knowledge and confidence and thus to improve their care.

Karen Forbes
April 2007

Part I

Pain in patients with cancer

2

Chapter 1

The principles of management of pain due to cancer

Karen Forbes

> **Key points**
> - Cancer pain may be due to the cancer itself, treatment of cancer or underlying illness.
> - Successful pain management requires a careful history, examination and relevant investigations.
> - A management plan should be agreed with the patient.
> - Patients require regular reassessment and access to support should their pain deteriorate.

1.1 Introduction

Pain is a feared complication of cancer with the vast majority of patients assuming that they will suffer from pain at some point in their illness when they receive a diagnosis of malignancy. A systematic review of pain over the last 40 years suggests that the prevalence of pain in all cancer patients remains high, and this prevalence varies according to the stage of the patient's disease. 33% of patients had pain following curative treatment and of patients having current active treatment 59% had pain, as did 64% of patients with advanced disease. The pooled prevalence of pain was over 50%, and over one third of patients graded their pain as moderate to severe. Thus, whilst it is not true that all patients with cancer will suffer from pain the majority do, and despite developments in pharmaceuticals and treatment approaches over the last 20–30 years, a significant proportion continue to live with moderate to severe pain. Successful pain management requires an understanding of the underlying mechanisms of cancer pain, careful clinical assessment, knowledge of treatment strategies and an ability to tailor them to the individual patient's changing needs.

1.2 **Neurophysiology of nociception**

Specialised sensory receptors sensitive to noxious stimuli (nociceptors) are present in connective tissues, skin, bone, muscle and viscera. Activation of these nociceptors conducts electrical discharges to the spinal cord. A-beta, A-delta and C sensory nerve fibres have a role in pain perception. A-delta fibres are thinly myelinated and rapidly conducting and are responsible for the sharp, stinging pain of acute injury. 'Polymodal' C fibres are unmyelinated and slower conducting and respond to a range of noxious stimuli producing a slow, dull, throbbing, more diffuse pain. These afferent fibres synapse with neurones within the dorsal horn of the spinal cord and, via interneurones, on to the thalamus and cortex. A-beta and other sensory fibres, also synapsing within the dorsal horn, may inhibit onward transmission; descending inhibitory neural pathways also have an inhibitory role, mediated via serotonin and noradrenaline. Opioid receptors are expressed on central and peripheral neurones; peripherally they are activated only in the presence of inflammation. They are responsible for inhibition of nociceptive neural pathways and thus in producing analgesia.

1.3 **Definition of pain**

The International Association for the Study of Pain defines pain as 'An unpleasant sensory and emotional experience associated with actual or potential tissue damage, or described in terms of such damage.' Others suggest 'Pain is whatever the experiencing person says it is, existing whenever the person says it does.' Whichever definition one chooses, it is important to remember that pain has both physical and affective components.

1.4 **Classification of pain**

Pain may be classified on the basis of neurophysiological mechanisms into somatic, visceral and neuropathic, or may be classified on a temporal basis.

Somatic or nociceptive pain occurs due to mechanical, thermal or chemical stimulation of nociceptors in skin, muscle, bone and associated connective tissues. It is described usually as aching and is well localised. Visceral pain occurs due to stimulation of nociceptors in thoracic, abdominal or pelvic viscera, often because of tumour infiltration or stretch, distortion or distension due to tumour mass. It has a deep pressure quality and is often poorly localised. Pain from intra-abdominal viscera may be referred to a distant skin surface, the classical example being shoulder tip pain secondary to diaphragmatic disease.

Neuropathic pain occurs secondary to disturbance of function or damage within the peripheral or central nervous system. It is often described as dull and aching, and may have associated areas of decreased or abnormal sensation. It may occur due to tumour infiltration or compression of central or peripheral nerves.

1.4.1 Temporal classification of pain

Patients with acute pain describe pain commencing over a defined, usually short, period of time, often associated with obvious physical signs and a physiological 'flight or fight' response. Such pain can occur in patients with cancer, for instance following a pathological fracture. Chronic pain is common in cancer and is defined as pain of more than 3 months duration. Patients adapt to chronic pain so that they no longer look pale with a tachycardia; indeed others may say they 'do not look as if they are in pain'.

Breakthrough pain, sometimes also known as episodic pain, is an exacerbation or increase of pain that occurs against a background of controlled pain, or pain of mild to moderate intensity. Drugs used to manage this pain are referred to as rescue or breakthrough medication.

1.5 Causes of pain due to cancer

Patients with cancer may have pain directly due to their disease process; as suggested above pain may occur due to tumour invasion or compression of normal tissues. Pain may also occur due to diagnostic or therapeutic interventions. In one survey, 78% of inpatients and 62% of outpatients had pain due to their cancer and about 20% had pain due to surgery, chemotherapy or radiotherapy. Up to 10% of pain may be due to non cancer factors such as associated comorbidities, although the prevalence of non-cancer-related pain does not appear to increase with age.

1.6 Clinical assessment of pain

In assessing a patient with pain it is necessary to take a careful pain history, to examine the patient and to order relevant investigations.

This will allow an assessment of the likely underlying cause and its association with the patient's disease state.

1.6.1 Elements of a pain history

- Site of pain.
- Quality of pain—character, abnormal sensations?
- Aggravating and relieving factors.

- Associated symptoms.
- Onset and duration.
- Response to previous medication.
- Impact on the patient's physical functioning.
- Impact on the patient psychologically.

Pain is both a physical and emotional experience and so the patient's thoughts and fears about their pain should be explored. The patient may be anxious, distressed or depressed about their pain, and their psychological state might explain why they have presented at that time or how they are responding to their current pain. Discussion should include what they think the current pain means and how it is affecting their life.

1.6.2 **Examination**

Careful physical examination should include a neurological examination and will be focused on looking for tenderness, deformity, organomegaly, areas of decreased or abnormal sensation and for associated muscle spasm, incoordination and difficulty with mobilising.

1.6.3 **Investigations**

It is good practice to order investigations, which are potentially inconvenient and uncomfortable for patients, only if they are likely to alter management. For patients with pain due to cancer, investigations should direct treatment, so that a radiograph of a painful long bone might indicate prophylactic pinning and radiotherapy, or a bone scan might suggest that radiotherapy for bone pain would be helpful.

1.7 **Discussing a management plan with the patient**

If cancer pain is to be managed successfully, the patient needs to be a partner in the management process. Patient and professional can agree on how the patient's pain should be managed, set realistic goals and plan when to assess whether these have been met and what would trigger reassessment or earlier intervention. This is particularly so if the patient is being asked to commence strong opioids (see Chapter 5). A management plan will include relevant treatments of the underlying disease, treatment with analgesics, consideration of non-drug measures such as heat, cold, immobilisation and complementary therapies and psychological support for the patient. Referral on to other agencies may be necessary and the patient should know who to contact should their pain worsen.

1.8 **Reassessment**

For some patients a carefully discussed pain management strategy may fail to improve their pain. This may be because the patient has been reluctant to use drugs as suggested, because they have not yet received an adequate dose, or because their underlying disease is progressing. In many patients, prognosis is limited and so prompt control of pain is extremely important. Patients need to be reassessed regularly and frequently enough to achieve and maintain pain control, even in the face of progressive disease.

1.9 **Summary**

Pain in patients with cancer may be due to the cancer itself, to diagnostic or therapeutic interventions for the cancer or due to underlying illness. Successful pain management requires knowledge of the possible underlying causes of cancer pain, taking a thorough history and examining the patient, arranging relevant investigations to identify the cause of the pain and treat where appropriate, and agreeing a management plan with the patient. In patients whose prognosis is often short and whose disease is progressing, frequent and regular reassessment will be necessary.

Key references

Foley, K.M. (1979). Pain syndromes in patients with cancer. In *Advances in pain research and therapy*, Vol. 2. International Symposium on Pain in Advanced Cancer (ed. J.J. Bonica and V. Ventafridda), pp. 59–76. Raven Press, New York.

International Association for the Study of Pain Subcommittee on Taxonomy (1986). Classification of chronic pain. *Pain* (Suppl. 3), 216–21.

McCaffery, M. (1968). *Nursing practice theories related to cognition, bodily pain and man-environment interactions*. University of California, Los Angeles.

Portenoy, R.K., and Hagen, N.A. (1990). Breakthrough pain: definition, prevalence and characteristics. *Pain*, **41**, 273–82.

Van den Beuken-van Everdingen, M., de Rijke, J., Kessels, A., Schouten, H., van Kleef, M. and Patijn, J. (2007). Prevalence of pain in patients with cancer: a systematic review of the past 40 years. *Ann. Oncol.* (epub ahead of print).

Part II

Treatment of cancer pain

Chapter 2

The range of treatments for pain due to cancer

Peter Hoskin

Key points

- Cancer pain will comprise a complex clinical picture often including a number of individual pains each with a somatic source and a variable but significant affective component requiring careful detailed assessment for each patient.
- The mainstay of management will be analgesics used according to the principles of the analgesic ladder but these should be augmented by appropriate adjuvant drugs such as non-steroidals, anxiolytics and antidepressants and for neuropathic pain, in particular, antidepressants and anticonvulsants.
- Non-drug treatments including acupuncture, transcutaneous electrical nerve stimulation (TENS), massage and supportive psychotherapy may have a major role in selected patients.
- Whenever possible specific anticancer treatment should be considered to address the underlying cause of the pain. Knowledge of the primary tumour and details of previous treatment will inform options for systemic treatment with chemotherapy or hormone manipulation.
- Radiotherapy has a major role in the management of bone metastases, cerebral metastases and pain due to progressive local tumour infiltration.
- Surgery for pathological fracture, vertebral collapse and bowel obstruction, and stenting for oesophageal, bronchial, ureteric and superior vena cava obstruction should also be considered.

2.1 **Introduction**

Pain due to cancer will primarily arise as a result of the growth, spread and local infiltration of a malignant tumour. Pain may be localised in one site, for example severe myofascial pain in the head and neck region from progressive tumours of the oropharynx or more widespread, typified by the picture of multiple bone metastases. The full range of available treatments should be considered for each patient and will include both non-specific pain modifying treatments and specific tumour modifying treatments. Selection of appropriate treatment for an individual must be on the basis of a careful and detailed appraisal of each individual's symptoms against a background knowledge of their underlying tumour and its past treatment.

2.2 **Pain modifying treatments**

2.2.1 **Pharmacological management**

The mainstay of pain management will, in most patients, be based on the analgesic ladder and the following chapters will consider in some depth the role of the ladder and, in particular, the use of opioid drugs. The majority of patients will require a strong opioid at some point but this is rarely sufficient alone.

In terms of analgesic management it is important to recognize the role of adjuvant analgesics, that is, drugs which do not themselves have intrinsic analgesic activity but which will modify the disease processes causing pain. When used in conjunction with an opioid analgesic they may substantially enhance pain relief and in some circumstances reduce opioid requirements. Examples of these drugs are shown in Table 2.1. Optimal use of these drugs requires careful pain assessment as discussed in the preceding chapter.

2.2.2 **Non-pharmacological management**

Alongside drug therapy non-pharmacological interventions should also be considered. It is important not to underestimate the role of simple psychological supportive measures since it is well recognized that cancer pain has a significant affective component due to the emotions of anger, depression, despair, fear and anxiety which accompany the scenario of advanced cancer. All measures will work better in an environment of hope, sympathy and empathy with treatment undertaken against a background of careful reassurance, realistic goals and close monitoring. Up to 30% of patients may have clinical depression or anxiety requiring more specialist intervention, both pharmacological and non-pharmacological, using appropriate psychological tools. Other interventions may also enhance pain relief,

Table 2.1 Adjuvant analgesics		
Drug	Action	Clinical indications
Non-steroidal anti-inflammatory drugs (NSAIDs)	Anti-inflammatory	Musculoskeletal pain Soft tissue pain
Anxiolytics	Anti-anxiety	Anxiety and agitation
Antidepressants	Antidepressant Nerve sedative	Depression Neuropathic pain
Anticonvulsants	Nerve sedative	Neuropathic pain
Corticosteroids	Anti-inflammatory	Hepatic pain Neuropathic pain Cerebral metastases
Antibiotics	Anti-infective	Cellulitis Infected tumour Abscess
Bisphosphonates	Osteoclast inhibition	Bone metastases

for example, the use of relaxation therapy, hypnotherapy, massage and acupuncture. Simple measures such as the direct application of heat pads or ice packs can be of value. The importance of careful reassurance with realistic goals, perhaps negotiating a lifestyle change to reduce activities which stimulate pain, particularly for the patient with troublesome incident pain, may also be valuable.

Specific neurolytic procedures may also have their role particularly with intractable neuropathic pain when spinal opioids or specific nerve root or plexus blocks may be invaluable. Specific examples would include coeliac plexus blockade for intractable pancreatic pain and caudal block for severe sacral pain.

2.3 Specific antitumour treatment in the management of cancer pain

2.3.1 Oncological treatment

Chemotherapy and radiotherapy have a fundamental role in symptom control and hence an integrated approach to the management of advanced cancer is essential with close interaction between oncologists and specialists in palliative medicine. Patients with advanced cancer may present a complex multifactorial constellation of symptoms but fundamental to the whole process is the underlying malignant condition and all opportunities for disease modification should be considered in order to achieve optimal pain control.

Radiotherapy is a locoregional treatment ideal for situations where the pain is due to local tumour infiltration, in particular, bone metastasis and soft tissue metastasis, and also where brain metastases causing raised intracranial pressure are responsible for intractable

13

headache. The primary tumour may also cause local pain and in many circumstances palliative radiotherapy will be of significant value in achieving useful pain control. Examples include tumours of the head and neck region, non-small cell lung cancer and carcinoma of the oesophagus.

Chemotherapy and hormone therapy are systemic treatments which do not target specific sites but, when effective, will result in generalized tumour control and potentially offer the most effective means of controlling multisite symptoms, for example, pain from multiple bone metastases.

The choice between chemotherapy and radiotherapy is related to the probability of response and the symptom profile. It is further influenced by the probability of significant toxicity, an issue which is usually more prominent in the use of chemotherapy than radio-therapy or hormone therapy. It is, however, important to note that there is good evidence to suggest that patients will often be prepared to accept significant treatment toxicity for only a small likelihood of improvement and such treatment options should not be denied without a full and frank discussion of these issues with the patient.

One of the major limitations of chemotherapy in this setting is the limited sensitivity of the common tumours to chemotherapeutic intervention, but with the development of new agents, for example, vascular targeting drugs and monoclonal antibody therapy, the range of treatment options is becoming wider and the availability of second, third and fourth line chemotherapy schedules is increasingly common. Examples are shown in Table 2.2. The decision to introduce chemo-therapy, radiotherapy or hormone therapy may be based on the following considerations:

1. Origin of pain and spatial distribution: radiotherapy will be better for local pain and systemic radiation in the form of radioisotope therapy or wide field radiotherapy may be better for scattered bone pain. Symptoms in the face of widespread metastatic disease however may benefit from the introduction of chemotherapy, often alongside radiotherapy for the local pain.

2. The probability of response, which will be based upon the primary histological type of the tumour, and also previous exposure to therapy.

3. Toxicity profile of the proposed intervention and patient acceptance of that degree of toxicity.

4. Performance status: patients with ECOG performance status 0 or 1 are most likely to benefit from the introduction of chemotherapy. Those with worse performance status, unless directly related to a readily reversible consequence of the tumour, will rarely do so.

Table 2.2 Chemotherapy options in advanced common solid tumour types

Tumour	First line	Second line	Third line
Breast	FEC	Taxotere ±herceptin*	Capecitabine
Colorectal	FOLFOX ±Bevacizumab	FOLFIRI	FOLFIRI/Cetuximab
NSCLC	Cisplatin/Gemcitabine	Taxotere	Pemetrexed
SCLC	Etoposide/Cisplatin	CAV	
Prostate (Hormone resistant)	Taxotere		
Pancreas	Gemcitabine		
Bladder	Cisplatin/Gemcitabine	MVC	

FEC = 5FU, epirubicin, cyclophosphamide; FOLFIRI = 5FU, folinic acid, irinotecan;
FOLFOX = 5FU, folinic acid, oxaliplatin; MVC = methotrexate, vinblastine, cisplatin;
CAV = cyclophosphamide, doxorubicin, vincristine;
NSCLC = non small cell lung cancer;
SCLC = small cell lung cancer,
* Herceptin in Her2 receptor positive patients only

5. Accessibility to preferred treatment: hormone therapy may be easily administered with simple outpatient medication; chemotherapy may require complex support and infrastructure with access to supportive intervention in the event of complications such as neutropenic sepsis.

2.3.2 **Surgery**

Surgery should not be excluded from the treatment options under consideration. In specific scenarios it will offer the quickest and most effective means of pain control. Examples include internal fixation of a long bone fracture in a mobile patient, kyphoplasty or fixation for vertebral collapse or bowel diversion in localised obstruction.

2.3.3 **Other interventions**

Interventional endoscopy and radiology have an increasing role enabling stent insertion as a relatively simple day case procedure. Examples include palliation of pain due to oesophageal or tracheal obstruction, superior vena cava obstruction or obstructive hydronephrosis.

Examples of common scenarios in the patient with advanced cancer and the possible treatment interventions are shown in Table 2.3.

2.4 **Summary**

Fundamental principles of pain control based on careful assessment and identification of the cause of pain, with appropriate treatment individualized on the basis of these findings, is paramount. There is a wide range of treatment options to be considered which will include both non-specific pain modifying therapy based on regular analgesia, adjuvant analgesics and other pain relieving measures, together with appropriate psychological support. Alongside this the role of specific tumour modifying treatment, either radiotherapy, chemotherapy or hormone therapy should always be included in the management options for cancer pain.

Table 2.3 Common painful clinical scenarios and available specific treatment interventions in advanced cancer				
Clinical condition	Treatments to be considered			
	Radiotherapy	Chemotherapy	Hormone Rx	Other
Bone metastases				
Local pain	All cases			
Widespread pain	All cases	Breast, lung, myeloma	Prostate, breast	Bisphosphonate
Pathological fracture	If inoperable or post op			Surgical fixation
Vertebral collapse	If inoperable or post op			Surgical fixation
				Balloon kyphoplasty
Cerebral metastases				
Solitary	Post op or radiosurgery			Surgical resection
Multiple	All cases	Germ cell, lymphoma, breast, SCLC		
Hepatomegaly	If large and not chemo responsive	All responsive tumours (see Table 2.2)	Breast, prostate, uterus	Corticosteroids
				Embolisation
				Radiofrequency ablation
Pelvic recurrence (cervix, rectum)	If no previous RT	Cervix colorectal		Caudal block
Head and neck tumour (local infiltration)	If no previous RT	Consider		Consider palliative resection
Chest pain from NSCLC	All cases	All cases		

Key references

Eisenberg, E., Berkey, C.S., Carr, D.B., Mosteller, F. and Chalmers, T.C. (1994). Efficacy and safety of nonsteroidal anti-inflammatory drugs for cancer pain: a meta-analysis. *J. Clin. Oncol.*, **12**, 2756–65.

Galbraith, S.M. and Duchesne, G.M. (1997). Androgens and prostate cancer: biology, pathology and hormonal therapy. *Eur. J. Cancer*, **33**, 545–54.

Hoskin, P.J. and Brada, M. (2001). Radiotherapy for brain metastases, consensus statement. *Clin. Oncol.*, **13**, 91–4.

Sze, W.M., Shelley, M.D., Held, I. , Wilt, T.J. and Mason, M.D. (2003). Palliation of metastatic bone pain: single fraction versus multifraction radiotherapy—a systematic review of randomised trials. *Clin. Oncol.*, **15**, 345–52.

Wong, R. and Wiffen, P.J. (2002). Bisphosphonates for the relief of pain secondary to bone metastases. *Cochrane Database Syst Rev*, (2) CD002068.

Chapter 3

The development and efficacy of the WHO analgesic ladder

Augusto Caraceni and Stefan Grond

Key points

- Use of the WHO analgesic ladder can control pain due to cancer for the majority of patients.
- The ladder is based on simple principles such as
  - simplicity in the choice of analgesic;
  - simplicity in the choice of route;
  - individualization of dose, particularly of strong opioids;
  - continuous pain requires continuous medication;
  - use of adjuvant analgesics;
  - treatment of adverse effects to allow adequate dose titration.
- The priniciples of the WHO ladder should be applicable in all care settings.
- While there are no randomized controlled trials (RCTs) of the method, these would now be impossible as it is accepted as the gold standard worldwide.

3.1 WHO ladder and WHO method for cancer pain relief

The 'WHO method for cancer pain relief' first published in the book *Cancer Pain Relief* by the World Health Organization (WHO) is now commonly referred to as the WHO analgesic ladder. The analgesic ladder was initially but one part of a broader number of recommendations designed to improve cancer pain, ranging from excellent assessment to pharmacological and non-pharmacological approaches. The sequential pharmacological approach to pain, with its emphasis on morphine used by mouth, by the clock, by the ladder was the core message heralding a powerful cultural change to the heterogeneous clinical practice common at that time.

The WHO method was developed as a universal clinical guideline that needed to be applicable throughout the world, it therefore needed to be simple and to include therapeutic options that were potentially available to all.

3.1.1 **Historical and cultural background**

The WHO initiative on cancer pain grew out of contributions from a number of clinicians, mainly pain experts working between 1950 and 1980, who were the foundation of a new specialty in pain and palliative care. At that time, pain was emerging as a subject of study and of clinical interest. The acceptance of pain, in particular chronic pain, as a disease state in its own right led to the development of a number of important concepts that continue to influence our clinical practice today:

- The patient's subjective experience as a focus of research and clinical interest.
- Pain as a multidimensional construct which require not only anaesthetic interventions, but multicomponent pharmacological and non-pharmacological strategies.
- Opioids as fundamental to the management of cancer pain despite the prejudices and fears about the use of opioids then prevalent.

Concurrent with these developments, clinicians were developing appropriate research methodologies, assessment tools and related statistical methods, particularly at the Memorial Sloan Kettering Cancer Centre in the USA, for investigating pain and its management. Morphine and other opioids were studied and equianalgesic conversion tables established, many of which are still in use today.

3.1.2 **The Milan WHO meeting**

The International Association for the Study of Pain was founded in 1973. Important congresses on cancer pain in Florence and then in Venice followed, where current experts shared their emerging clinical experience rejecting the current wisdom of primary recourse to nerve blocks and invasive procedures and favouring a new approach where analgesics were the first choice of treatment and invasive procedures second or last resource.

In 1982, these congresses led on to the WHO initiative, bringing together a number of eminent clinicians to design a strategy to develop a worldwide approach to cancer pain relief. The WHO guidelines represented a consensus of expert views, based on the clinical experience within a developing field.

3.1.3 **The demonstration project**

The WHO programme had two main objectives:

- The publication of a guideline to be disseminated and used for educational and political efforts to develop the field and improve the control of cancer pain.
- The conduct of two demonstration studies to show that the guidelines had a clinical impact. Study 1 was an observational study of the practice of treating cancer pain in centres which were not exposed to the WHO method. Study 2 was assessing the same data but in centres applying the draft interim WHO guidelines.

The WHO demonstration studies indeed showed that pain was better controlled when applying the WHO method compared with the level of pain relief obtained by centres not exposed to the method, but lack of statistical sophistication and insufficient researcher confidence led to a relatively understated publication, which might otherwise have been one of the most significant analgesic studies of the last 20 years.

The success of the programme was enormous considering the limited resources on which it was based, in that the WHO ladder is now considered the gold standard for comparing any new approach. No studies since have addressed the issue of tackling cancer pain with the same vision and scope, or with the same policy impact, as that achieved by the WHO method (Figure 3.1).

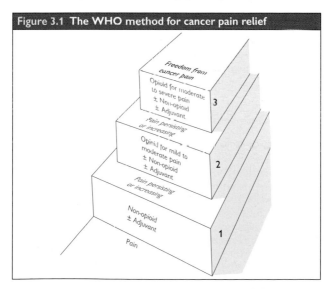

Figure 3.1 The WHO method for cancer pain relief

Freedom from cancer pain

Opioid for moderate to severe pain ± Non-opioid ± Adjuvant **3**

Pain persisting or increasing

Opioid for mild to moderate pain ± Non-opioid ± Adjuvant **2**

Pain persisting or increasing

Non-opioid ± Adjuvant **1**

Pain

Figure 3.1 is reproduced with kind permission from the World Health Organization (WHO) ▣ www.who.org

Although there are no randomized control trials proving its efficacy, the WHO analgesic ladder is widely accepted throughout the world and has been implemented through many national guidelines. Critics argue the efficacy of the analgesic ladder has been evaluated in only three major clinical studies. Proponents counter that these studies involved over 5000 patients and that randomized controlled trials of a method adopted as the gold standard would now be impossible.

3.2 Validation studies

Ventafridda *et al.* (1987) performed a 2-year retrospective study in 1229 patients. In 71% of these patients the WHO analgesic ladder provided adequate pain relief without requiring neurolytic procedures. Of these patients, 97 were treated only at step I (non-opioids), 210 only at step II (weak opioids), 231 only at step III (strong opioids) and 292 required all three steps of the ladder. Adjuvant drugs were added in 79% of patients. The mean pain scores fell to about one-third of the initial intensity and remained low until death. The most frequent adverse events were dry mouth, drowsiness, constipation, sweating and nausea and vomiting.

Zech and colleagues (1995) assessed 2118 cancer patients in a 10-year prospective study over a period of 140 478 treatment days. The patients had been referred to a specialist cancer pain unit. Forty-one per cent of patients were followed up until death. Step I was used in 11%, step II in 31% and step III in 49% of treatment days. Co-analgesics and adjuvants to treat other symptoms were administered on 37% and 79% of days, respectively. In addition, palliative anticancer treatment was performed in 42% and nerve blocks in 8% of patients. The percentage of patients with severe pain was reduced from 78% to 13% after 1 week and to 7% in the last days of life. Over the whole treatment period, good pain relief was reported in 76%, satisfactory efficacy in 12% and inadequate efficacy in 12% of patients. Other clinical symptoms were likewise reduced, with the exception of neuropsychological symptoms. The latter were the major symptoms on 23% of days, followed by nausea, constipation and anorexia.

Mercadante (1999) enrolled 3678 patients in a palliative home care programme into a prospective study over a 9-year period. Therapy was required for 70% of patients. In the last week of life, 16%, 49%, and 35% of patients were on steps I, II and III, respectively; 16% of patients required parenteral administration. Adjuvant drugs were given if needed. A minority of patients (3%) underwent invasive procedures. The mean pain intensity (0–10) was reduced from 4.4 at referral to 2.5 after 1 week and 2.3 in the final week of life. The intensity of nausea and vomiting, dry mouth, drowsiness, constipation and confusion increased during the course of treatment.

3.2.1 **Level of evidence**

All major validation studies and several small studies confirm that the WHO analgesic ladder provides adequate analgesia in 70–90% of cancer patients. Jadad and Browman (1995) have, however, criticised the value of these studies, because they have no control group, hence they suggest that the level of evidence is insufficient.

The WHO method for cancer pain relief was published in 1982, well before the use of guidelines was prevalent. A comparison with contemporaneous or historical controls could have been performed 20 years ago, but would not be possible today, because cancer pain treatment all over the world has been influenced by the WHO analgesic ladder. The WHO analgesic ladder has stood the test of time as an effective and feasible approach and remains the gold standard for cancer pain management. In order to improve this gold standard in the future, the efficacy and feasibility of new concepts and modifications of the ladder must be investigated in (preferably randomized) controlled trials.

3.3 **Possible directions for future research**

There is increasing debate about the usefulness of step II of the ladder. Several studies have demonstrated no advantage in using weak opioids or even disadvantages in comparison to using low doses of strong opioids. Therefore, it is becoming more common to omit step II and to start with low doses of morphine in opioid-naïve cancer patients (Mercadante, et al. 1996). It is believed that weak opioids only have advantages in societies where patients and medical practitioners are reluctant to use morphine. The most frequently used weak opioid is codeine, which is a prodrug of morphine, however, the increasing worldwide availability of tramadol may reopen the discussion on step II (Grond, et al. 2004).

The discussion on the use of the second step of the ladder is mostly an academic one and does not negate the usefulness of the WHO analgesic ladder. 'Attention to detail' and 'for the individual' are important elements of the WHO analgesic ladder. If non-opioids provide no adequate pain relief, patients should be commenced on opioids. Depending on individual factors (patient, disease, society) the medical practitioner will then choose to start weak opioids or low doses of strong opioids.

Many other aspects of the efficacy of the WHO analgesic ladder are of interest and should be investigated in controlled studies, however, most clinicians argue we should not question the efficacy of the WHO analgesic ladder in principle; it is more important to optimize and improve the concept and to concentrate limited resources on offering effective pain relief to the numerous patients who still continue to receive inadequate analgesia.

Key references

Grond, S. and Sablotzki, A. (2004) Clinical pharmacology of tramadol. *Clin. Pharmacokinet.,* **13**, 879–923.

Houde, R.W., Wallenstein, S.L. and Beaver, W.T. (1965). Clinical measurement of pain. In *Analgesics* (ed. G. de Stevens), pp. 75–122. Academic Press, New York.

Jadad, A.R. and Browman, G.P. (1995). The WHO analgesic ladder for cancer pain management. Stepping up the quality of its evaluation. *JAMA,* **274**, 1870–3.

Mercadante, S. (1999). Pain treatment and outcomes for patients with advanced cancer who receive follow-up care at home. *Cancer,* **85**, 1849–58.

Mercadante, S., Porzio, G., Ferrera, P., Fulfaro, F., Aielli, F., Ficorella, C., et al. (1996). Low morphine doses in opioid-naïve cancer patients with pain. *J. Pain Symptom Manage.,* **31**, 242–7.

Seymour, J., Clark, D. and Winslow, M. (2005). Pain and palliative care: the emergence of new specialties. *J. Pain Symptom Manage.,* **29**, 2–13.

Ventafridda, V., Caraceni, A. and Gamba, A. (1990). Field-testing of the WHO guidelines for cancer pain relief. In *Advances in pain research and therapy,* vol. 16. 2nd International Congress on Cancer Pain (ed. K.M. Foley, V. Ventafridda, and J.J. Bonica), pp. 451–64. Raven Press, New York.

Ventafridda, V., Tamburini, M., Caraceni, A., DeConno, F. and Naldi, F. (1987). A validation study of the WHO method for cancer pain relief. *Cancer,* **59**, 851–56.

World Health Organization (1986). *Cancer pain relief.* World Health Organization, Geneva.

Zech, D., Grond, S., Lynch, J., Hertel, D. and Lehmann, K.A. (1995) Validation of World Health Organization Guidelines for cancer pain relief: a 10-year prospective study. *Pain,* **63**, 65–76.

Part III

Opioids in cancer pain

Intruduction to Part 3: Opioids in Cancer pain

Since the original publication of the World Health Organization analgesic ladder, an updated version has been published which refers to opioids at the second and third steps of the ladder in a slightly different way.

Opioids at the second step of the ladder, referred to as step II in this book, were originally known as 'weak' opioids, but are now defined as 'opioids for mild to moderate pain'. Opioids at the third step of the ladder, referred to as step III in this book, were originally known as 'strong' opioids, but are now defined as 'opioids for moderate to severe pain'. In this book the simpler phrases 'weak' and 'strong' opioids are retained.

Chapter 4

Opioid receptors

Catherine E. Urch

Key points

- There are four members of the opioid receptor family mu, delta, kappa and ORL-1.
- G protein linked receptors.
- Acute response to ligand binding differs from chronic response.
- Acute response includes dimerisation, endocytosis and inhibition of adenylyl cyclase, cAMP systems and hyperpolarization of the neuron.
- Chronic response includes altered G protein, adenylyl cyclase proteins, increased phosphorylation, receptor modulation, rectification of hyperpolarization and attenuation of extreme inhibition.
- New altered receptor activation and cell inhibition state achieved.
- Polymorphisms in receptor and enzyme pathways give insight into inter-individual response.

4.1 Introduction

There are three main subtypes of opioid receptor, namely, mu, delta and kappa; a more recent addition is the opioid receptor like (ORL-1) or orphanin receptor. The mu, delta and kappa receptors are very similar sharing over 70% sequence homology, whilst the ORL-1 receptor shares only 50% sequence homology. Extensive pre-mRNA splicing gives rise to numerous splice-variants. The mu receptor gene has been shown to have 25 different splice variants in mice, 8 in rats and 11 in humans, which are controlled by diverse promoters. It has been demonstrated that different splice variants exhibit differences in agonist induced G protein activation, adneylyl cyclase activity and receptor internalisation. Further modifications may lead to differences in phosphorylation, membrane translation, scaffolding protein binding and G protein binding. These modifications extensively alter the potential activation and destination of the receptor.

4.2 **Endogenous ligands**

The three families of endogenous opioid peptides are well characterized. They are the endorphins, enkephalins and dynorphins, which have binding affinities to all three receptors. Each family derives from a distinct gene, their precursors being pro-opiomelanocortin, proenkephalin and prodynorphin. The selective mu ligand endomorphins do not have an identified precursor. Peripherally they interact extensively with immune cells, primarily in inflammatory states, when beta-endorphin containing cells as well as signalling molecules (vascular P-selectin and intercellular adhesion molecule-I (ICAM-1)) are upregulated.

4.3 **The receptor family**

4.3.1 **Role of delta opioid receptor**

Evidence suggests that other opioid endogenous ligands and receptors are linked to analgesic response and to mu receptor activation, for instance deletion of the delta receptor gene and pre-proenkephalins inhibits the development of morphine tolerance, but not withdrawal, in mice. The potency of mu agonists is increased by the co-administration of delta agonist, which also induces a translocation of delta receptors to the cell surface. Delta receptors are involved in analgesia, but may also be linked to seizures, and response to ischaemia.

4.3.2 **Role of kappa opioid receptor**

Kappa receptors are also involved in analgesia, in particular in response to inflammation (peripherally), however, activation produces a number of unpleasant side effects centrally, such as nausea and vomiting, dysphoria and a diuresis due to negative regulation of antidiuretic hormone (ADH).

4.3.3 **Role of ORL-1 receptor**

The ORL-1 receptor was identified because of its homology with classical opioid receptor types. Its natural ligand is known as 'nociceptin' or 'orphanin'. Centrally ORL-1 agonists appear to oppose mu opioids, for example, binding by buprenorphine leads to limitation of action at mu receptors, and knockout orphanin mice show a lack of tolerance to morphine. The ORL-1 receptor is involved in modulation of a range of biological functions including the stress response, movement, memory, cardiovascular and renal functions.

4.4 **The mu opioid receptor**

This is clinically the most important of all the receptor family and will be discussed in more detail. It is the main opioid receptor responsible for inhibition of nociceptive neural pathways, and is exploited by all exogenous opioids (Figure 4.1).

4.4.1 Expression

The mu receptor is expressed on central and peripheral neurones, although in the latter it is only activated in response to inflammatory stimuli. Peripherally mu receptors are found pre- and post-synaptically, for example in the dorsal horn; approximately 70% are expressed on the primary afferent terminations (pre-synaptic) modulating the input. Mu receptors are present on C and A delta fibres, the sympathetic nervous system and immune cells. Centrally they are expressed widely including the cerebral cortex, the amygdala and the peri-aquaductal grey. In the peri-aquaductal grey, the presence of mu receptors on inhibitory neurones leads to disinhibition of descending pathways resulting in excitation, as opposed to the more usual result of inhibition of neural transmission. The relative contribution of each binding site to the overall analgesic effect of systemic opioids has not been investigated. The receptor undergoes pre- and post-transcriptional splicing and alteration, leading to a huge variation in the activation state of the receptor.

4.4.2 Intracellular activation and signalling pathways

The opioid receptors belong to the superfamily of seven transmembrane-spanning G protein coupled receptors. Their primary function is to transmit extracellular stimuli to intracellular signals. Opioid receptors are transduced by the G_i/G_o proteins which are relatively resistant to tolerance or desensitisation. This causes inhibition of adenylyl cyclase, reduction of cyclic AMP, suppression of tetrodotoxin-resistent sodium channels and activation of Na^+/K^+ ATPase. Opioids induce membrane hyperpolarization as a result of increased potassium rectifying currents (centrally) and inhibition of voltage dependent calcium channels (peripheral and dorsal horn neurones). In addition, opioid receptor activation increases the release of intracellular calcium stores; the mechanism is not fully understood.

Opioid receptors and the accompanying G proteins interact with a vast array of other intracellular proteins responsible for trafficking receptors to membrane, anchoring and scaffolding proteins, all of which in turn alter the response of the receptor to a ligand. G protein coupled receptors, including mu, kappa and delta receptors have been shown to form dimers, homo- and hetero-oligomers, which have relevance in internalisation and activation pathways. Dimerisation modulates receptor pharmacology which could present targets for novel interventions.

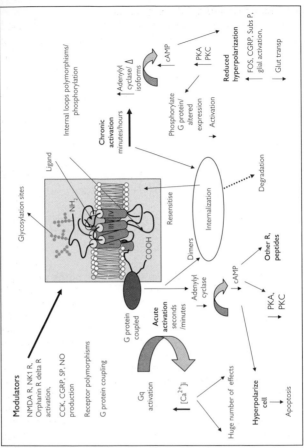

Figure 4.1 A schematic summary of some of the consequences of mu opioid receptor activation. The central cartoon of the opioid receptor illustrates its transmembrane regions, the extra-cellular N terminal and intracellular C terminal, binding of a ligand as well as sites for modulation. The receptor is coupled to a G protein, the activation and phosphylation of which determines the consequence of ligand binding. Acute and chronic activation summaries are illustrated. Chronic mu opioid receptor activation leads to alterations which modulate the intense hyperpolarization of the neurone and a new activation state is achieved.

4.4.3 **Modulation of opioid responses**

There are multiple cellular adaptations in response to chronic opioid exposure, which may lead to tolerance. Nociceptive tolerance to exogenous opioids is relatively easy to produce in animal studies, where repeated doses of a given opioid rapidly lead to loss of efficacy in response to noxious stimuli. However, in humans tolerance to respiratory depression, nausea, vomiting and sedation have all been widely reported, tolerance to constipation is not seen and to analgesic efficacy is debated. There does not appear to be a simple correlation between exposure to opioids and induction of analgesic tolerance in humans, rather a process of adaptation occurs which may also depend on many other factors.

Cellular processes which occur in response to chronic ligand binding to mu receptors include diminution of spare opioid receptors, decreased receptor density, altered coupling, activation and phosphorylation of G proteins and alteration of downstream pathways (such as upregulation of adenylyl cyclase isoforms, cAMP/cAMP dependent protein kinase (PKA) and mitogen-activated protein (MAP) kinases). This upregulation correlates negatively with the activity of Na^+/K^+ ATPase (which is impaired in chronic morphine exposure), can induce cellular apoptosis in experimental spinal cord preparations and causes downregulation of glial glutamate transporters. It has been reported that chronic exposure to mu or delta agonists induces and upregulates the pro-excitatory peptides calcitonin-gene-related peptide (CGRP) and substance P and protein kinase C (responsible for phosphorylation). The effect of these adaptations is to lead to a pro-excitatory state and an attenuation of the inhibitory effects of opioid activation.

Other modulatory responses include the altered expression of peptides. Alterations in the glutamate (N-methyl-D-aspartate (NMDA)) or substance P binding sites (NK1 receptors) affect the development of tolerance and the reinforcing properties of morphine, respectively. Endogenous peptides such as neuropeptide FF, cholecystokinin, nociceptin and dynorphin exhibit anti-opioid actions, which in turn modulate the physiological action and outcome of opioid agonists. Chronic morphine exposure leads to little change in mu receptor expression, but more extensive alteration in arrestin, GRK, NMDA and gamma amino butyric acid (GABA) and heat-shock protein 70 transcription (which may help protect against opioid induced apoptosis). In addition there are changes in the non-neuronal population of glial cells, with increased activation in response to chronic morphine exposure.

4.5 **Receptor activation versus endocystosis**

Increased acute uncoupling of mu receptor from active G proteins, mediated by phosphorylation, is followed by arrestin binding and internalisation of the receptor. The receptor is then either degraded or recycled to the cell surface, the process being conceived as a resensitisation rather than a desensitisation. The process is modulated by second messenger linked proteins such as protein kinase C (PKC) or A (PKA), interactions with G protein coupled receptor kinases, scaffolding proteins, and arrestin. Internalisation of opioid bound receptors is also dependent on the opioid and cell type.

These acute desensitisation processes may be a protective mechanism whereby cells adapt to avoid physiological tolerance by attenuating receptor response to a new sustainable level. Drugs such as morphine, which induce less receptor internalisation, produce more rapid and sustained tolerance in animal studies, but a cell specific response may contribute to determining the physiological actions of opioids *in vivo*. The use of combinations of opioids is becoming more common in clinical practice, clinicians citing putative differences in receptor activation versus endocystosis (RAVE), the formation of dimers and oligomers and the resulting G protein cascade reactions. However, given the complex, cell specific and multi-feedback dimension of opioid interactions, it is probably simplistic to assume that greater benefit from using such combinations might outweigh other factors such as poor patient compliance and prescriber dosing errors.

4.6 **Pharmacogenomics and the opioid system**

Clinically there are large interindividual responses to pain and analgesics. As discussed above receptor and peptide responses all modulate the clinical efficacy of exogenous opioids. Recently the role of genetic diversity of receptors, messenger systems, and drug metabolism pathways in altering the clinical response to opioids have been investigated. Despite a huge array of described genetic polymorphisms only a few have accumulated any evidence of potential importance in modulating pain therapy; these include the mu opioid receptor, catechol-O-methyl transferase (COMT), melanocortin-1 receptor (MC1R), cytochrome P450 2D6 (CYP2D6) and P-glycoprotein (ABCB1), all of which affect the action of morphine, codeine, tramadol or morphine-6-glucuronide (M6G). The functional importance of one variant of the mu opioid receptor has been reported (where an asparagine is substituted for aspartate coded for by a single nucleotide polymorphism 118Adenine > Guanine). Studies suggest that patients with this polymorphism needed more alfentanil post-op and achieved less analgesia, and homozygotes required significantly more morphine than heterozygotes. Overall it is suggested that the 118G polymorphism decreases opioid potency by a factor of 2–3. While the molecular consequences of the polymorphism meant a two-fold reduction in receptor transcription was suggested, the binding of morphine, other ligands and secondary messenger system activation was found to be unaffected.

The COMT variation 472G>A polymorphism leads to reduced function of the enzyme, less degradation of dopamine, and depletion of enkephalin, with a secondary up-regulation of mu receptors and an increased efficacy of morphine. Seventy-five per cent of MC1R variants are red-headed pale skin phenotypes, with two important polymorphisms, 451C>T and 478C>T, which result in loss of receptor function. These phenotypes have a more active kappa opioid system and greater response to pentazocine and morphine. The CYP2D6 polymorphism is more widely reported, and non-functioning mutations are found in 7% Caucasians, resulting in reduced or no analgesia from codeine or tramadol.

So far the clinical consequences of uncovering genetic polymorphisms are restricted to explaining the efficacy of codeine. The study of mutations affecting opioid receptors, activation, ligand response and pain processing are of great interest, but with as required analgesia and switching between opioids they may help to explain interindividual effects but do not alter clinical therapy.

4.7 **Opioid antagonists**

Naloxone (short-acting) and naltrexone (long-acting) are opioid antagonists and block mu, delta and kappa receptors equally. They are generally only used to reverse respiratory depression associated with opioid overdose as they will also reverse analgesia.

4.8 **Summary**

As can be seen from the above discussion, opioids, the receptors, activation state, secondary messenger pathways and response to endogenous and exogenous ligands form a vast array of interconnecting networks all of which have subtle bearings on each other and all other neural interactions. Reducing the actions of a ligand to merely binding affinities or any one action is to belittle a magnificent pathway, the true complexity of which is only now being understood. It should thus not be surprising that not all patients respond to pain, pain processing or opioids in the same way.

Key references

Bailey, C.P. and Connor, M. (2005). Opioids: cellular mechanisms of tolerance and physical dependence. *Curr. Opin. Pharmacol.*, **5**, 60–8.

Davis, M.P., LeGrand, S.B. and Lagman, R. (2005). Look before leaping: combined opioids may not be the rave. *Support. Care Cancer*, **13**, 769–74.

Lotsch, J. and Geisslinger, G. (2006). Current evidence for a genetic modulation of the response to analgesics. *Pain*, **2**, 1–5.

Milligan, G. (2005). Opioid receptors and their interacting proteins. *Neuromolecular Med.*, **7**, 51–9.

Mollereau, C., Roumy, M. and Zajac, J.M. (2005). Opioid modulating peptides: mechanism of action. *Curr. Top. Med. Chem.*, **5**, 341–55.

Watkins, L.R., Hutchinson, M.R., Johnston, I.N. and Maier, S.F. (2005). Glia: novel counter-regulators of opioid analgesia. *Trends Neurosci.*, **28**, 661–9.

Zollner, C. and Stein, C. (2006). Opioids. *Handb. Exp. Pharmacol.*, **177**, 31–63.

Chapter 5

Starting opioids for moderate to severe pain: talking to the patient

Karen Forbes and Colette Reid

Key points

- Patients and professionals have inappropriate fears about morphine.
- Patients' fears must be explored before they are offered morphine.
- Tolerance, addiction and serious adverse effects such as respiratory depression are not relevant in clinical practice.
- Ongoing professional education is necessary to improve pain control in patients with cancer.

5.1 Introduction

Analgesic drugs are the mainstay of the management of pain due to cancer. The World Health Organization (WHO) analgesic ladder provides a simple method by which a majority of patients' pain can be controlled. If patients are on regular, full dose opioids at step II of the ladder, with non-steroidal anti-inflammatory drugs (NSAIDs) if they are indicated and the patient can take them, and adjuvants if they are indicated, then the method dictates the patient should commence opioids for moderate to severe pain at step III of the ladder. Unfortunately, some patients' pain management is hindered by patient, carer and, at times, health professionals' concerns regarding the use of morphine. These include worries about addiction, likelihood of serious adverse effects and tolerance. In addition, for the patient and their carers, there is often the psychological significance of commencing morphine. It is important that these issues are addressed in order to overcome reluctance to opioid therapy to allow effective pain relief.

There are a number of barriers to patients receiving adequate pain control. These can be divided into attitudes and beliefs, knowledge deficits and clinical practices and laws and regulations. In some parts of the world, morphine and other strong opioids are not available still, in others excessive bureaucracy surrounds prescribing these drugs. It is noteworthy that the amount of morphine used in those countries where prescribing limits are not imposed and bureaucracy is low is far higher than where these restrictions apply.

5.2 **Attitudes and beliefs**

Both patients' and professionals' attitudes and beliefs about strong opioids, and morphine in particular, can hinder patients achieving pain control. The attitudes and beliefs are similar, but they may be expressed in different ways. These attitudes and beliefs include addiction, tolerance, morphine not being a very effective drug, being appropriate only for the dying and morphine having either euphoric or serious, unmanageable and life-threatening side effects.

5.2.1 **Addiction**

Studies suggest that professionals believe that patients given morphine to manage pain due to cancer will become addicted to it, however, they are not reluctant to prescribe morphine in patients with cancer pain, presumably reasoning that it does not matter if the patient is addicted if they have a short prognosis. Unfortunately, this attitude is responsible for many non-cancer patients with chronic pain being denied a trial of opioids. Many patients are also reluctant to commence morphine as they do not wish to become addicted.

Without a past history of dependence on drugs or alcohol, psychological dependence on medically prescribed opioids is extremely rare. If pain is controlled by other means (e.g. nerve blocks or tumour-specific treatment such as radiotherapy), then the dose of morphine may be reduced or even withdrawn without any resulting adverse psychological consequences. Physical dependence can occur, however. If morphine therapy is ceased abruptly, some patients may suffer flu-like withdrawal symptoms. These symptoms are managed easily by more gradual withdrawal of opioids over a few days.

5.2.2 **Tolerance**

Tolerance describes the need to take increasing doses of drug for a given effect. Both patients and professionals assume that patients' opioid doses will need to increase over time to maintain pain relief. Patients often express this by saying 'I don't want to take it yet doctor, I'll save it until I really need it', however, many patients remain on stable doses of opioid for weeks or even months. Whilst a very few patients seem to develop some tolerance to the analgesic effects of opioids (often those patients using a parenteral route), in the majority the need for a dose increase is normally due to disease progression. Tolerance is not relevant in routine clinical practice.

5.2.3 **Morphine's efficacy**

There are some patients and professionals who believe morphine and other strong opioids are not good analgesics, but they are used in patients with cancer pain because they make people feel better; the assumption being they make patients euphoric. A 'high' is undoubtedly sought by people misusing opioids, however clinical practice suggests patients taking opioids, particularly at too high a dose, are drowsy, slowed up and muddled and universally find the sensation unpleasant.

As long as patients have opioid responsive pain, morphine is a good analgesic, with no ceiling dose and no other alternative opioid has yet been demonstrated to be more effective.

5.2.4 **Adverse effects**

Many patients are justifiably worried about side effects when commencing strong opioids. Their worries need to be explored and predictable side effects such as constipation, nausea and vomiting anticipated and managed prophylactically (see Chapter 7).

5.2.4.1 *Sedation and driving*

Patients should be warned they will feel drowsy on commencing or increasing the dose of morphine, but this should wear off over 3–5 days once their dose is stabilized. Patients on stable doses of morphine drive as well as age and sex matched controls, and patients should be told they can drive once they have been on a stable dose of morphine for 3–5 days.

5.2.4.2 *Hallucinations and confusion*

Many patients have had experiences of friends or relatives on morphine becoming confused or hallucinating, often some years ago, and are concerned about these side effects for themselves. They should be reassured confusion and hallucinations may occur if the dose needs to be escalated rapidly, but these side effects can be managed and if necessary switching to a different opioid might produce a better side effect profile. Professionals should know that confusion and hallucinations need to be managed rather than being accepted as inevitable.

5.2.4.3 *Respiratory depression*

Professionals are often reluctant to use opioids in patients with chronic lung disease because they fear respiratory depression. Provided morphine dose is titrated carefully against pain, significant respiratory depression does not occur. A retrospective case note analysis by Thorns and Sykes (2000) failed to show any correlation between strong opioid use in the last week of life and increased incidence of sudden death or difference in the description of death. Pain stimulates respiration and this antagonises the central respiratory depressant effects of morphine. Although morphine reduces the sensitivity of the respiratory centre to pCO_2, the peripheral receptors responsible for hypoxic drive and the medullary centres regulating cardiovascular behaviour are unaffected, allowing compensation.

5.3 The psychological impact of being offered morphine

Severe pain is more common as cancer progresses and the recommendation that a patient begins treatment with morphine often has a significant psychological impact. Popular culture suggests that morphine is used only for patients who are very ill and dying and patients will protest that they are not 'at that stage yet'. Often they are reluctant to tell friends and relatives that they have been offered or have commenced morphine because this will cause their loved ones worry or distress.

5.4 Talking to patients

In an important qualitative study Reid (2007) talked to patients as they commenced step III opioids about their thoughts and fears. Patients talked about morphine as 'the last resort before dying'. They thought the doses of morphine they needed would have to be increased, but contrary to professionals' previous interpretation of this as being an understanding of tolerance, patients meant their doses would have to be increased as their disease progressed. Many felt this would inevitably hasten their death, but accepted this as the only way their pain could be controlled as they became more ill. These are important findings with implications for clinical practice and clearly need corroborating in further studies, but should guide us in our discussions with patients as we offer them therapy with morphine.

Patients' fears and expectations need to be explored, but they should be reassured that they are being offered morphine because of the severity of their pain, rather than the stage of their disease, that side effects will be anticipated and managed, morphine does not become a less effective analgesic with time and there is no evidence that morphine used properly hastens death. Many patients find it helpful to hear that if their pain could be abolished by a nerve block, for example, they would be able to discontinue its use over a few days without adverse effect. Professionals need to be alert to their patients' anxieties, whilst developing familiarity and comfort with morphine as an effective and safe step III analgesic.

5.5 Professionals' knowledge and attitudes

The literature suggests that professionals have poor knowledge about opioid prescribing and mistaken attitudes about tolerance, addiction and efficacy. Education can improve knowledge and attitudes but there is no evidence thus far that this results in improved prescribing practice and patient care. Those familiar with the use of opioids in patients with cancer pain have a duty to challenge and educate their colleagues so that the principles of the WHO analgesic ladder can be properly and fully implemented to provide improved pain control in patients with cancer, which we know can be achieved.

Key references

Elliott, T. and Elliott, B.A. (1992). Physician attitudes and beliefs about the use of morphine for cancer pain. *J. Pain Symptom Manage.*, **7**, 141–8.

Elliott, T.E., Murray, D.M., Elliott, B.A., Braun, B., Oken, M.M., Johnson, K.M., et al. (1995). Physician knowledge and attitudes about cancer pain management: a survey from the Minnesota cancer pain project. *J. Pain Symptom Manage.*, **10**, 494–504.

Reid, C. (2007). Cancer pain and the World Health Organization analgesic ladder. MD thesis. University of Bristol, unpublished.

Thorns, A. and Sykes, N. (2000). Opioid use in last week of life and implications for end-of-life decision-making. *Lancet*, **356**, 398–9.

Vainio, A., Ollila, J., Matikainen, E., Rosenberg, P. and Kalso, E. (1995). Driving ability in cancer patients receiving long-term morphine analgesia. *Lancet,* **346**, 667–70.

Chapter 6

Principles of opioid titration

Marie Fallon and Sandra McConnell

Key points

- There is great variation in the dose of opioid required by individual patients.
- Doses must be tailored to the individual's need and should start low and then be adjusted (titrated) according to response—up or down.
- Short acting opioids should be used during the initial titration period and then converted to longer acting formulations when the required dose to achieve pain control is reached.
- Opioids are useful for neuropathic pain.
- Adjuvants have an important role in controlling some types of pain where opioids give insufficient analgesia or where adverse effects become intolerable.

6.1 Introduction

Opioids are unlike most other medications in that there is no standard dose: the dose must be tailored to the individual's response. Opioid titration is the process whereby the dose of opioid analgesic is altered until the minimum dose which controls an individual's pain is reached or intolerable toxicity develops.

6.2 Titration of opioids

Titration is necessary when a patient is first commenced on an opioid and also when pain intensity, in a patient already receiving an opioid, changes. Titration can thus involve an increase or decrease in dose. Generally, normal release oral morphine is used for initial titration. Normal release morphine acts within 20–30 min and lasts 4 h. It is therefore prescribed 4-hourly. The same dose which is prescribed 4-hourly is also prescribed 'as required' for breakthrough pain.

Breakthrough pain has been defined by Portenoy and Hagen (1990) as a 'transitory increase in pain to greater than moderate intensity (that is, to an intensity of "severe" or "excruciating") which occurs on a baseline pain of moderate intensity or less (that is, no pain or pain of "mild" or "moderate" intensity)'. The administration of 'as required' medication may be repeated 4-hourly if necessary as the peak plasma level generally occurs after 60 min (with the exception of methadone—see below). Regular review of the 'as required' medication a patient has used will guide titration: within 24 h, steady state of normal release morphine would have been reached. Thus every 24–48 h, the total opioid requirement from the preceding 24 h can be divided by six to obtain the new 4-hourly and 'as required' dose. This process continues until pain is relieved, at which point the opioid is usually converted to a modified release preparation. This is also known as 'controlled release' morphine. Normal release morphine (usually one-sixth, but can be as low as 5% of the total daily dose) should still be available for breakthrough pain. Sometimes, normal release morphine is administered prophylactically for activities which are recognized to cause exacerbations of pain in an individual. Generally this should be 30 min before the activity if taken by the oral route. This is usually an acceptable way of managing pain in patients who have well controlled background pain (on modified release morphine) and in whom it would be impossible to titrate opioid dose high enough to control breakthrough pain without causing intolerable adverse effects.

Monitoring of 'as required' normal release morphine use continues to guide further titration: the total 24 h dose required being converted to modified release morphine accordingly (unless, of course, requirements have increased as a result of a transient event, for example, an investigation/long journey or normal release morphine is being used prophylactically for prevention of movement related pain or another predictable, transient event).

6.2.1 **Moving from step II to III opioids**

If a patient has pain sufficiently severe to merit progression from step II to III of the World Health Organization (WHO) analgesic ladder, it is important to ensure that the initial dose of strong opioid (also known as opioid for moderate to severe pain) prescribed has greater analgesic effect than the step II weak opioid (also known as opioid for mild to moderate pain), for example, a patient receiving 60 mg codeine 6-hourly is already receiving the equivalent of 36 mg of morphine per day. Thus the 4-hourly dose of oral morphine in this case would be 6 mg. In such circumstances, 10 mg would usually be prescribed unless the patient is frail, elderly or has renal dysfunction. If it is decided to commence strong opioid therapy in someone who is opioid-naïve, generally a 10 mg oral dose should be used initially and then titrated according to response.

6.2.2 Titration using non-oral routes

The principles of titrating opioids given by alternative routes are similar to those for oral morphine. Patients can either start with small dose subcutaneous boluses every 4 h (often via a butterfly needle to prevent frequent injections) or commence a continuous subcutaneous infusion with boluses as required for breakthrough pain. Once again, the total dose of drug needed during the preceding 24 h guides adjustment in the 4-hourly or infusion dose.

6.2.3 Titration of methadone

Methadone titration is more complicated than titration of morphine and the alternative opioids in view of its very different pharmacokinetics. Its plasma half-life varies dramatically between individuals (from 8 to over 100 h), making accumulation and resultant toxicity, including severe respiratory depression, a potentially serious drawback. For this reason it should be used only under specialist supervision.

6.2.4 Dose reduction

A patient's opioid dose may need to be titrated downwards in the event of pain reduction, for example, due to antitumour therapy, local anaesthetic or neuroablative procedures. A trial of dose reduction may also be warranted where pain is controlled and adverse effects are troublesome.

6.3 Opioid responsiveness

Some pain syndromes are more opioid responsive than others. In particular, nociceptive pain is more responsive than neuropathic pain. However, although it is frequently claimed that neuropathic pain is opioid unresponsive, it often does respond to opioids. Unfortunately, the dose required to control pain in these circumstances may be higher than can be tolerated by the patient, because of the resulting adverse effects.

6.3.1 Opioid titration in neuropathic pain

Moderate to severe neuropathic pain should be managed similarly to any other pain of that intensity. Opioids should be titrated as described above. In many patients with comorbidity, such as cardiac or renal disease, opioids may actually be the safest analgesic if chosen and titrated carefully. Although it is thought that methadone may be the opioid of choice for neuropathic pain due to its N-methyl-D-aspartate (NMDA) receptor antagonistic effect and its powerful agonist effect at mu and delta opioid receptors, its superior effect has not yet been proven.

In circumstances where adverse effects limit opioid titration, analgesia may be improved by the addition of co-analgesics and/or adjuvant medication, which may be opioid sparing, that is, a reduction in opioid dose may be possible.

Co-analgesics are non-opioid analgesics which can be combined with opioids, for example, paracetamol or non-steroidal anti-inflammatory drugs (NSAIDs), and which may allow a smaller dose of opioid to be administered.

6.4 **The role of adjuvants**

Adjuvant drugs are medications which are principally meant for a use other than analgesia but which can have a pain relieving effect in particular situations. These drugs can be added at any step of the WHO analgesic ladder and include tricyclic antidepressants, anticonvulsants, corticosteroids, anaesthetic agents, antispasmodics, muscle relaxants and bisphosphonates.

6.4.1 **Tricyclic antidepressants and anticonvulsants**

The adjuvant drugs most commonly used for neuropathic pain are tricyclic antidepressants and anticonvulsants. Corticosteroids, anaesthetic agents and antiarrhythmics are also sometimes used.

There is little difference in effectiveness between tricyclic antidepressants and anticonvulsants (number needed to treat is approximately 3 in both cases) and no evidence that either is more helpful than the other in treating pain in which certain neuropathic symptoms predominate. Often the choice of drug is guided by the potential adverse effects for an individual patient and cost. Occasionally both classes of drug are prescribed concurrently although it is best to optimize the dose of the first before introducing the second.

6.4.1.1 *Adverse effects*

Typically tricyclic antidepressants cause adverse effects including dry mouth, constipation, urinary retention, postural hypotension, drowsiness, blurred vision and confusion. They may also result in cardiac arrhythmias. Although not licensed for neuropathic pain, tricyclics such as amitriptyline are used regularly. The usual starting dose is 25 mg at night (10 mg if frail or elderly) and this is titrated every 5–7 days according to response up to approximately 75 mg. Anticonvulsant drugs can cause somnolence, dizziness and cerebellar signs such as ataxia, tremor, nystagmus and diplopia. Gabapentin and the newer drug pregabalin are licensed for neuropathic pain and are generally felt to be better tolerated. Despite this, doses are still required to be increased gradually.

6.4.2 **Other approaches for neuropathic pain**

Corticosteroids are limited in their usefulness due to their adverse effects with prolonged use. Ketamine is an intravenous anaesthetic which can be effective in neuropathic pain treatment (unlicensed indication) when given in sub-anaesthetic doses. It is given either intramuscularly or, occasionally, intravenously in palliative care and acts as an NMDA antagonist to exert its analgesic effect. Unfortunately, its use is limited by adverse effects: it causes increased blood pressure (and is, therefore, contraindicated in those with uncontrolled hypertension), tachycardia and psychotomimetic effects. Haloperidol is frequently co-administered to reduce hallucinations. Benzodiazepines can be used as an alternative to haloperidol. Lidocaine, a local anaesthetic, is useful in anaesthetic interventions, however, intravenously it should be used only with careful evaluation of response and in the specialist setting with appropriate cardiac monitoring.

In up to 10% of patients with neuropathic pain, spinal analgesia or a neurolytic procedure may be required to give adequate pain relief. Non-drug treatments such as transcutaneous electrical nerve stimulation (TENS) should also be considered.

6.5 **Summary**

If patients have pain which is not controlled on regular, full dose, step II opioids they should be commenced on step III opioids. Best practice is to titrate to pain control using normal release opioids, and then to convert patients to more convenient modified release preparations. Patients will require active management of adverse effects to allow adequate dose titration. Adjuvant drugs can be added at all steps of the WHO analgesic ladder. Some pain syndromes may be more responsive to opioids than others, but a trial of opioids is worthwhile since response cannot be predicted.

Key references

Cherny, N.I., Thaler, H.T., Friedlander-Klar, H., Lapin, J., Foley, K.M., Houde, R., et al. (1994). Opioid responsiveness of cancer pain syndromes caused by neuropathic or nociceptive mechanisms: a combined analysis of controlled, single-dose studies. *Neurology*, **44**, 857–61.

Mercadante, S., Porzio, G., Ferrera, P., Fulfaro, F., Aielli, F., Ficorella, C., et al. (2006). Low morphine doses in opioid-naïve cancer patients with pain. *J. Pain Symptom Manage.*, **31**, 242–7.

Nicholson, A.B. (2004). Methadone for cancer pain. *Cochrane Database of Syst. Rev.*, **2**, CD003971.

Portenoy, R.K. and Hagen, N.A. (1990). Breakthrough pain: definition, prevalence and characteristics. *Pain*, **41**, 273–81.

Portenoy, R.K., Foley, K.M. and Inturrisi, C.E. (1990). The nature of opioid responsiveness and its implications for neuropathic pain: new hypotheses derived from studies of opioid infusions. *Pain*, **43**, 273–86.

Chapter 7

Management of adverse effects

Marie Fallon and Sandra McConnell

Key points

- Opioids may cause CNS, GI, autonomic and cutaneous adverse effects.
- Adverse effects must be differentiated from comorbid conditions and drug interactions.
- Opioid adverse effects may be treated by decreasing dose of opioids, opioid switching, changing the route of administration and/or symptomatic management.
- Opioid toxicity must be screened for and treated without delay.

7.1 Introduction

Although opioids are often very effective analgesics, like most drugs they are not without adverse side effects. Effective cancer pain management involves maximising the analgesic effect whilst minimizing adverse effects. Approximately 10–30% of cancer pain patients have either excessive adverse effects, inadequate analgesia or both.

In order to minimize the adverse effects of opioids, it is necessary to be able to identify and manage them. Ideally, common preventable adverse effects should be anticipated and treated prophylactically.

7.2 Adverse effects of opioids

Adverse effects commonly associated with opioid therapy can be divided into four groups:

- Central nervous system (CNS) effects: including drowsiness, cognitive impairment, hallucinations, vivid dreams, peripheral shadowing of vision, delirium, agitation, euphoria, myoclonus, hyperalgesia, seizure disorder and respiratory depression.
- Gastrointestinal (GI) effects: including constipation, nausea and, less commonly, vomiting.

- Autonomic: including dry mouth, urinary retention and postural hypotension.
- Cutaneous: including itch and sweating.

Following initiation of opioid therapy, or an increase in dose, some adverse effects manifest for a while before settling spontaneously. Nausea occurs in up to two-thirds of patients but frequently resolves after 3–4 days. Sedation and cognitive impairment also improve frequently after 5–7 days. This is in contrast to constipation which affects almost all patients on opioid drugs and does not abate with time.

7.3 **Patient susceptibility to adverse effects of opioids**

Several factors influence the likelihood of opioid adverse effects:

- Genetic variability affects sensitivity to opioid analgesia and is probably equally important in determining predilection to adverse effects, for example, by affecting drug metabolism.
- The degree of responsiveness of the pain to opioid analgesia— some pains, such as neuropathic pain, are more difficult to control with opioids, requiring higher doses to be administered.
- Prior exposure to opioids—tolerance to some adverse effects develops with time. Patients who have had previous exposure are generally less prone to sedation or respiratory depression, however, delirium and myoclonus tend to be the more prominent CNS effects in this setting.
- Rate of titration of the dose—rapidly escalating doses give little time for tolerance to develop to adverse effects. In particular, hyperalgesia has been associated with rapid increases in opioid dose.
- Route of administration—there can be reduced nausea and vomiting with subcutaneous (and perhaps rectal) administration of opioids and reduced constipation in some cases with transdermal fentanyl compared with oral morphine (although this could be due to differences in drug rather than route).
- Concomitant medication—some drugs, for example, tricyclic antidepressants, some anticonvulsants, benzodiazepines and antibiotics may cause adverse effects which are additive or synergistic to those of opioids by altering their absorption, metabolism or clearance.
- Renal function—if renal function is impaired there may be reduced clearance of active metabolites such as morphine-6-glucuronide (M6G). Renal function reduced by more than 2 standard deviations (SDs) from the mean was associated with an increased chance of morphine adverse effects in a recent retrospective study.

- Hepatic function—there is only slight reduction in clearance of morphine as a result of mild to moderate hepatic impairment but severe decline in function may cause more noticeable reduction in elimination. Retrospective analysis has shown that poor hepatic function (>2 SD above the mean) is correlated with higher incidence of morphine intolerance.

- Age of patient—elderly patients require lower doses of opioid to manage their cancer pain and this is important to bear in mind, as they are at higher risk of opioid toxicity. An age over 78 years has been associated with increased risk of morphine adverse effects.

- Haematological indices—a white cell count (WBC) $>7 \times 10^9$ mmol/l and platelet count $>210 \times 10^9$ mmol/l have been found to be associated with greater chance of morphine adverse effects in a recent retrospective study and, hopefully, this will be investigated further in the future.

In general there is little evidence to suggest that any one opioid has an appreciably better adverse effect profile than any other.

7.4 Comorbidity

In patients receiving opioid therapy symptoms and signs may develop, imitating opioid-induced adverse effects, which are actually a consequence of comorbid conditions or drug interactions. Approximately 80% of patients with advanced cancer experience severe pain but it is not uncommon for these patients to have other problems such as sepsis, hypercalcaemia, or cerebral/leptomeningeal metastases causing sedation, cognitive impairment, nausea and vomiting. Similarly renal or hepatic failure may produce myoclonus in addition to the above symptoms and signs. Bowel obstruction, antibiotics, chemotherapy or radiotherapy could also cause nausea and vomiting. Dehydration, hyponatraemia, hypoxia, cerebrovascular accident, extradural haemorrhage or drugs such as benzodiazepines or tricyclic antidepressants may also result in sedation and cognitive impairment. It is very unusual for patients receiving stable opioid doses to suddenly develop adverse effects and comorbidity (particularly renal impairment) or drug interactions must be sought to explain the change in condition.

Drugs which interact with opioids can be found in Appendix 1 of the British National Formulary (BNF).

7.5 Strategies for managing adverse effects

Assuming that adverse effects are indeed attributable to opioid therapy they can be managed by

- Reducing the dose of opioid.

- Ensuring adequate hydration.
- Switching route of administration.
- Symptomatic management of specific adverse effects.
- Opioid switching (also known as opioid rotation or substitution).

7.5.1 **Dose reduction**

If pain is adequately controlled, reducing the opioid dose by 25–50% usually reduces adverse effects of mild to moderate intensity (especially CNS effects). Sometimes the addition of a non-opioid co-analgesic or adjuvant analgesic may be helpful in allowing opioid dose reduction whilst maintaining analgesia, however, both have the potential to cause adverse effects imitating those of the opioid, which may confuse the clinical picture. Specific antitumour therapies, such as radiotherapy or chemotherapy, regional anaesthetics or neuroablative procedures may also have an opioid-sparing effect thus facilitating dose reduction.

7.5.2 **Hydration**

As many opioids are renally cleared, adequate hydration and mainte-nance of renal function are helpful in eliminating excess drug and/or metabolites. This may require administration of parenteral fluids if, for example, the patient is unable to take oral fluids due to drowsiness or confusion.

7.5.3 **Route of administration**

Sometimes a change in route of administration can help alleviate adverse effects, for example, changing from oral to subcutaneous opioid may improve nausea and vomiting. Similarly, myoclonus may be reduced in patients on subcutaneous morphine compared to those using the oral route. Where CNS toxicity persists and/or pain is still uncontrolled despite optimization of systemic analgesia, chang-ing to spinal (epidural or intrathecal) administration of opioid, with or without local anaesthetic or clonidine, often has a beneficial effect on the balance between analgesia and adverse effects. However, this is a more invasive option and, like all invasive procedures, is dependent on the skill of the operator for its success.

7.5.4 **Symptomatic management**

Recommendations for symptomatic management of adverse effects are largely empirical or derived from anecdotal experience as there are few studies examining this area. This may, at least in part, be due to the difficulty of distinguishing pure opioid effects from comorbidity and other drug effects.

Although drug management of adverse effects is not ideal given the problems of polypharmacy (increased numbers of medications for those already taking multiple drugs, reduced compliance, risk of further adverse effects or interactions), sometimes it allows pain control to be achieved. Where possible, the different options for dealing with each individual situation should be discussed and patient preferences should be considered when deciding on the optimum management.

7.5.4.1 Constipation and nausea and vomiting

Constipation occurs in 40–70% of patients whose chronic cancer pain is treated with oral morphine. As with most adverse effects, comorbid conditions and other drug therapy may worsen this situation. In view of the high incidence of this symptom and its poor correlation with dose of opioid, laxatives should be prescribed prophylactically in conjunction with opioids to try to prevent constipation. Usually a stool softener and a stimulant laxative are required. Opioid-induced nausea and vomiting frequently ease a few days after initiation of therapy, however, in 15–30% of patients, nausea persists. Antiemetics are selected on the basis of the inferred mechanism of nausea (chemoreceptor trigger zone), for example, haloperidol or metoclopramide; the latter also for gastric stasis.

7.5.4.2 Sedation

Sedation affects 20–60% of cancer patients receiving regular oral morphine. Psychostimulants have been tried with good effect but, as these agents can themselves cause significant adverse effects (hallucinations, delirium, psychosis and tachycardia) they are not routinely used. Delirium is frequently managed with neuroleptics (haloperidol particularly) and if coupled with agitation, a benzodiazepine is added. Baclofen, benzodiazepines such as diazepam, clonazepam and midazolam, valproate and dantrolene sodium have all been used in the symptomatic management of myoclonus. Pruritis as a consequence of opioid therapy, which occurs in ≥ 10% of those on longterm oral morphine, is generally managed with antihistamines or paroxetine (unlicensed indication).

7.6 Opioid switching

Opioid switching (or rotation) involves changing from one opioid to another and may be necessary especially when pain is uncontrolled and/or adverse effects persist despite the measures described above. In more than half of patients with chronic pain and inadequate response to one opioid, there is clear improvement in their condition as a consequence of opioid switching. Predominant adverse effects/level of analgesia have been reported to improve in approximately 70% of cases of change in opioid. It may be beneficial to switch opioid in up to 40% of patients and sometimes multiple changes of drug are required (hence the term opioid rotation). The choice of which drug to switch to is largely based on anecdotal evidence or clinical experience as there is no robust evidence to imply that any one agonist is appreciably better than its alternatives. Pure opioid agonists such as oxycodone, methadone, hydromorphone, and fentanyl are advised. It should be noted, however, that drugs such as fentanyl and methadone take time to reach therapeutic plasma concentrations and are, therefore, not the best first alternatives in cases of uncontrolled pain.

7.6.1 **Conversion ratios**

Although doses of the alternative opioid are guided by conversion ratios there is significant interindividual variability in analgesic response to any particular opioid as a consequence of genetic polymorphism and variation in receptor affinities for each opioid. These factors result in what is known as incomplete cross-tolerance (Table 7.1).

Table 7.1 Generally accepted conversions	
PO morphine: SC or IV morphine	2:1 (–3:1)
PO morphine: SC diamorphine	3:1
PO morphine: SC alfentanil	30:1
PO morphine: PO oxycodone	2:1
PO morphine: PO hydromorphone	7.5:1
PO morphine: TD fentanyl	See manufacturer's dose (p. 145)
SC morphine: SC fentanyl	100:1

PO morphine: PO methadone—depends on previous dose of opioid and specialist help should be sought if considering a switch to this opioid

- If morphine 30–90 mg PO then use a ratio of 4:1
- If morphine 90–300 mg PO then use a ratio of 8:1
- If morphine >300 mg PO then use a ratio of 12:1
- If oral morphine dose was much more than 300 mg then ratio of >12:1 will be needed

PO = oral, SC = subcutaneous, IV = intravenous, TD = transdermal.

In view of the unpredictable effects of switching to another opioid, safe practice is to reduce the dose calculated using the conversion tables by 30–50% and then to titrate either up or down depending on response. This is of greater importance at higher doses where cross-tolerance can have a larger impact and it is wise to obtain specialist advice in this instance. However, regardless of the size of the dose of opioid being switched, it is vital that patients are observed closely during the conversion period.

7.7 **Summary**

Like most drugs, opioids have adverse effects; these are significant as they may limit dose titration and thus compromise control of pain.

A number of factors contribute to the patient's susceptibility to adverse effects; reversible factors should be managed where possible and other strategies such as ensuring adequate hydration and anticipating inevitable side effects such as constipation should be employed. Should patients develop intolerable adverse effects, then dose reduction, pharmacological management of side effects and switching to an alternative opioid should be considered.

Key references

Cherny, N., Ripamonti, C., Pereira, C., Davis, C., Fallon, M., McQuay, H., et al. (2001). Strategies to manage the adverse effects of oral morphine: an evidence-based report. *J. Clin. Oncol.*, **19**, 2542–54.

de Stoutz, N.D., Bruera, E. and Suarez-Almazor, M. (1995). Opioid rotation for toxicity reduction in terminal cancer patients. *J. Pain Symptom Manage.*, **10**, 378–84.

Expert Working Group of the European Association for Palliative Care. (1996). Morphine in cancer pain: modes of administration. *B.M.J.*, **312**, 823–6.

Hanks, G.W., Conno, F., Cherny, N., Hanna, M., Kalso, E., McQuay, H.J., et al. (2001). Morphine and alternative opioids in cancer pain: the EAPC recommendations. *Br. J. Cancer*, **84**, 587–93.

Mercadante, S. and Bruera, E. (2006). Opioid switching: a systematic and critical review. *Cancer Treat. Rev.*, **32**, 304–15.

Riley, J., Ross, J.R., Rutter, D., Shah, S., Gwilliam, B., Wells, A.U., et al. (2004). A retrospective study of the association between haematological and biochemical parameters and morphine intolerance in patients with cancer pain. *Palliat. Med.*, **18**, 19–24.

Part IV

Oral opioids

Chapter 8

Morphine

Marie Fallon and Sandra McConnell

Key points

- Morphine is considered the first line strong opioid for cancer pain and can be administered via different routes.
- Patients, carers and health care professionals' concerns regarding morphine must be addressed to allow successful pain management.
- Morphine is metabolized in the liver and is therefore susceptible to interactions with other drugs.
- Morphine metabolites are excreted by the kidney and may accumulate in renal impairment.
- Adverse effects of morphine may be managed by dose reduction, change in route of administration, opioid switching and/or symptomatic measures.

8.1 Background

Although opium has been used for many centuries, morphine was not isolated until 1804. The German pharmacist who discovered it named it 'morphium' after Morpheus the Greek god of dreams, but its name was later changed to end in '–ine' in keeping with the other alkaloids. In the past it was used as a remedy for opium and alcohol addiction as well as for the management of pain.

Today, the World Health Organization (WHO) analgesic ladder recommends strong opioids for the treatment of moderate to severe pain. While it has no demonstrated therapeutic benefit over alternative opioid agonists, oral morphine is used routinely as the first line treatment for cancer patients with this intensity of pain. Oral morphine's ready accessibility, ease of administration, proven efficacy and comparatively low cost when compared with its alternatives account for its frequent use for cancer pain relief. In addition, and importantly, it is the opioid with which health care professionals are most familiar.

8.2 **Concerns about morphine**

As discussed previously (see Chapter 5), patients, carers and professionals may have concerns about commencing strong opioids. Clinical experience suggests that these anxieties are most acute when patients are offered morphine. This is probably because morphine has been the opioid used most commonly for cancer pain in most countries, so that patients are aware of the drug and associate it with cancer and with care at the end of life. As for all strong opioids, patients' expectations and fears need to be discussed before they are offered morphine so that misconceptions and misunderstandings can be explored to enable patients to take the drug with confidence, thus increasing the likelihood of achieving good pain relief.

8.3 **Routes of administration**

Morphine can be administered by several different routes: oral, rectal, subcutaneous, intravenous (IV), epidural and intrathecal. Less commonly, it may be given intramuscularly, sublingually, or topically.

The oral route of administration is preferred due to ease of use and patient acceptability. When the patient is unable to swallow or absorb oral medication then other routes are employed. The route of administration may also be altered in the event of adverse effects and/or inadequate analgesia. It is estimated that approximately 25% of patients need a parenteral route of administration of opioid medication at some time in their illness.

When patients who are established on oral morphine develop swallowing or absorption problems, suppositories are an alternative for those who find the rectal route acceptable. If unavailable, normal release oral morphine may be administered rectally at the same dose, as the bioavailability is the same. The sublingual route is another option. In palliative care the subcutaneous route is preferred. A subcutaneous infusion via a device such as a small portable syringe driver is used commonly. In this instance, a half to one-third of the oral dose is infused. Subcutaneous boluses (one-sixth of the 24 h dose) may be given for breakthrough pain if required.

In patients with gastrostomy (PEG) tubes, liquid or suspensions of normal release or modified release morphine can be given.

The intravenous route is sometimes used for titration in pain crises to allow the dose of morphine required to be assessed more quickly. This route may also be used in patients who have established IV access or where subcutaneous administration is not possible, for example, in marked oedema, reduced peripheral circulation, coagulation disorders or where there are problems of erythema or swelling at the site of administration. Intramuscular morphine is rarely used in palliative care as it is more painful than the subcutaneous route. Morphine has also been applied topically to painful wounds such as pressure sores or fungating malignant lesions (usually mixed in gel) with good effect in many cases.

In situations where systemic analgesia has been optimized but pain remains uncontrolled, and/or adverse effects are problematic, the spinal route of administration (epidural or intrathecal) may be more successful. Local anaesthetic and/or clonidine may be added to improve the analgesic effect. As a guide, the oral morphine dose is divided by 10 to give the equivalent epidural dose and by 100 to yield the intrathecal dose.

8.4 **Pharmacokinetics**

Oral morphine has a highly variable bioavailability (15–60%). It undergoes substantial first pass metabolism when taken by mouth. A minimal amount of free morphine is excreted in the urine, bile or faeces. The drug is principally metabolized by the liver; UDP–glucuronosyl-transferase (UGT) and cytochrome P450 are the main enzymes involved. Natural variation in the genetic expression of these enzymes may explain part of the interindividual variability in dose requirements of morphine. In addition, the co-administration of some drugs may induce or inhibit morphine metabolism. Anticonvulsants such as carbamazepine, phenytoin, phenobarbital and some antibiotics (e.g. rifampicin) are enzyme inducers and expedite clearance of morphine. In contrast, tricyclic antidepressants and phenothiazines enhance morphine effects by interfering with its metabolism. In addition, benzodiazepines competitively inhibit glucuronidation of morphine and may intensify sedation, hypotension and delirium by their synergistic action. Morphine glucuronidation in patients with cancer pain is not affected by either the dose of morphine or the duration of treatment. Fortunately most patients with mild liver impairment are still able to tolerate oral morphine but for those with more severe disease, a reduction in dose and increased dosing interval are usually required.

8.4.1 **Morphine metabolites**
The major metabolites produced are morphine-3-glucuronide (M3G) and morphine-6-glucuronide (M6G). The main product, M3G, lacks analgesic activity and was thought to be responsible for some of the neurological adverse effects associated with morphine, however, evidence is mixed. M6G, on the other hand, is an active metabolite which is considerably more powerful than morphine in its analgesic activity: if morphine-6 beta-glucuronide is administered subcutaneously it is around twice as potent as morphine and, if administered intrathecally, it is approximately 650 times more effective than

morphine, however, morphine metabolites are rarely found intrathecally when morphine is given via this route due to lack of first pass metabolism. When morphine is given systemically, the M6G formed has low central nervous system (CNS) penetration.

8.4.2 **Morphine in renal disease and the elderly**

Morphine metabolites are eliminated by the kidneys, hence neurotoxicity may result from accumulation in cases of impaired renal function. Consequently, morphine should be prescribed with caution in such patients (by reducing the dose and/or increasing the dosing interval). In this circumstance, it may be more appropriate to use an alternative opioid, for example, fentanyl or alfentanil.

As a general rule, the elderly require lower doses of morphine than their younger counterparts with pain of similar intensity.

8.5 **Administration and formulation**

The WHO analgesic ladder dictates that analgesics should be given, 'by mouth', 'by the clock', 'by the ladder'. Oral morphine is the drug on which most of the evidence of the efficacy of the WHO analgesic ladder is based.

Oral morphine is available in both normal and modified release preparations. Normal release morphine's onset of action is generally 20–30 min with peak levels reached after approximately 60 min. When the correct dose for an individual patient's pain is achieved, its analgesic effect will last for approximately 4 h, making it ideal for titration (see Chapter 6). Commercially available formulations of normal release morphine include: Sevredol® scored tablets (10 mg (blue), 20 mg (pink) and 50 mg (pale green) tablets); Oramorph® oral solution (10 mg/5 mL); concentrated oral solution (100 mg/5 mL); and 10 mg/30 mg/100 mg unit dose vials. Some patients prefer or require liquid morphine but often dislike its bitter taste.

Once a stable dose of normal release morphine is reached it is advisable to convert to a modified release preparation, with a slower onset but longer duration of action for ease of administration and to maintain a more steady level of analgesia. In general, modified release preparations have an onset of action at 1.5 h with peak analgesic effect after 2–4 h and duration of action of either 12 or 24 h depending on the formulation. There are no generic modified release preparations. Since the pharmacokinetics of the different proprietary preparations of modified release morphine may vary slightly, it is recommended that patients are prescribed one modified release morphine preparation only. Should the brand they use need to be changed for some reason, then dosage requirements should be reviewed. Currently available preparations are given in Table 8.1.

Table 8.1 Preparations of modified release morphine

		MST continus®	MST continus®	Zomorph®	Morph-gesic® SR	MXL®
Formulation		Tablet	Suspension	Capsule enclosing pale yellow pellets	Tablet	Capsule
Dose interval		12 h	12 h	12 h	12 h	24 h
Dose available	5 mg	White	N/A	N/A	N/A	N/A
	10 mg	Brown	N/A	Yellow/clear	Buff	N/A
	15 mg	Green	N/A	N/A	N/A	N/A
	20 mg	N/A	✓	N/A	N/A	N/A
	30 mg	Purple	✓	Pink/clear	Violet	Light blue
	60 mg	Orange	✓	Orange/clear	Orange	Brown
	90 mg	N/A	N/A	N/A	N/A	Pink
	100 mg	Grey	✓	White/clear	Grey	N/A
	120 mg	N/A	N/A	N/A	N/A	Green
	150 mg	N/A	N/A	N/A	N/A	Blue
	200 mg	Green	✓	Clear	N/A	Red-brown
✓ = Dosage available; N/A = not available						

Patients may require a combination of individual tablets, for example, 50 mg – 2 × 20 mg + 1 × 10 mg.

Both Zomorph® and MXL® capsules can be swallowed whole or the capsules can be opened and the contents sprinkled onto soft food. The patient should have access to normal release morphine, at one-sixth of the total daily dose, for breakthrough pain and the modified release dose should be adjusted accordingly if more than two extra doses per day are required regularly. Although there is no upper dose limit for morphine, pain is controlled for most patients on less than 200 mg of oral morphine per day. While some patients with advancing disease need frequent alteration of their opioid dose as a consequence of escalating pain, most experience an interval of weeks, months or even longer where the dose remains stable or requires only minor alteration.

Morphine suppositories are available in 10, 15, 20 and 30 mg preparations.

Injectable morphine is available as 1, 2, 10, 15, 20 and 30 mg/mL solutions. Versions in combination with antiemetics are not recommended for use in palliative care since the ability to alter the dose of the opioid and the antiemetic independently is usually required. The oral to parenteral potency ratio of morphine is between 2:1 and 3:1.

8.6 **Regulations**

Prescribers should be familiar with the legal requirements regarding morphine which is a Class A controlled drug, subject to controlled drug regulations relating to prescriptions, safe custody and the need to keep registers. Morphine therapy also has implications for those wishing to travel abroad and prescribers should be aware of the legal requirements both for leaving the country carrying opioids (a doctor's letter or, currently, in the case of more than 1200 mg morphine being carried, a Home Office Licence) and for entering the country to be visited (need to contact the relevant Embassy, Consulate or High Commission for information—ideally written).

Key references

Anderson, G., Sjøgren, P., Hansen, S.H., Jensen, N.H., and Christrup, L. (2004). Pharmacological consequences of long-term morphine treatment in patients with cancer and chronic non-malignant pain, *Eur. J. Pain*, **8**, 263–71.

British National Formulary (2007). BMJ Publishing Group Ltd. http://www.bnf.org.uk/ accessed 4 March 2007.

Fukshanky, M., Are, M. and Burton, A. (2005). The role of opioids in cancer pain management. *Pain Pract.,* **5**, 43–54.

Paul, D., Standifer, K.M., Intrurrisi, C.E. and Pasternak, G.W. (1989). Pharmacological characterisation of morphine-6 beta-glucuronide, a very potent morphine metabolite. *J. Pharmacol. Exp. Ther.,* **251**, 477–83.

Snyder, S.H. and Pasternak, G.W. (2003). Historical review: opioid receptors. *Trends Pharmacol. Sci.*, **24**, 198–205.

Thorns, A. and Sykes, N. (2000). Opioid use in the last week of life and implications for end-of-life decision-making. *Lancet*, **356**, 398–9.

Vigano, A., Bruera, E. and Suarez-Almazor, M.E. (1998). Age, pain intensity and opioid dose in patients with advanced cancer. *Cancer,* **83**, 1244–50.

Chapter 9

Oxycodone

Colette Reid and Eija Kalso

> ### Key points
> - Oxycodone is a potent opioid analgesic.
> - It has an analgesic and side effect profile similar to morphine.
> - It is an alternative to morphine in patients with moderate to severe cancer pain with inadequate analgesia or unacceptable side effects due to morphine.

9.1 History and prescribing

Oxycodone has been in clinical use as an opioid analgesic since 1917 but until relatively recently was not widely used for cancer pain. Previously in the USA it had been considered as an opioid suitable for use at the second step of the World Health Organization (WHO) analgesic ladder, and so was manufactured in fixed dose combination preparations with aspirin or paracetamol. At the same time, it was used in parenteral formulations for the treatment of acute pain in Scandinavia as an opioid for moderate to severe pain. The confusion over its classification as either an opioid for mild to moderate pain or an opioid for moderate to severe pain arose from the early potency studies conducted in the USA by Beaver and colleagues that suggested when oxycodone was administered intramuscularly it was only two-thirds to three-quarters as potent as intramuscular morphine.

In the early 1990s the first randomized controlled studies were performed comparing intravenous patient controlled analgesia (PCA) titration and oral (solution) oxycodone and morphine in cancer pain by Kalso and colleagues (1990). These studies showed that these two opioids had comparable efficacy and adverse effect profiles. The efficacy of oral, intravenous, rectal and subcutaneous oxycodone in cancer pain was confirmed by other groups and oxycodone was shown to produce only weak spinal analgesia.

Purdue Pharmaceuticals developed a modified release formulation of oxycodone which was compared with morphine in several sponsored studies on cancer-related pain. These randomized controlled trials confirmed that oxycodone was as useful as morphine and demonstrated wide variations in equianalgesic dose ratios from 1:1 to 1:2.3. Oxycodone was thought to be less likely to cause hallucinations or nightmares and vomiting in these studies. Oxycodone was subsequently relaunched in modified and normal release formulations suitable for use in chronic pain. It is currently available in the UK in modified release tablet, normal release capsule and liquid and parenteral formulations under the trade names OxyContin® and OxyNorm®.

9.2 **Basic pharmacology**

The pharmacology of oxycodone is not as well defined as one would expect, given that it has been in use for so long. Oxycodone (14-dihydrohydroxycodeinone) is a semisynthetic derivative of thebaine. Oxycodone is a selective mu opioid receptor agonist like morphine with very little binding to either delta or kappa opioid receptors. It has been shown to have an abuse liability profile consistent with full mu opioid receptor agonism. However, its affinity at the mu opioid receptor is significantly lower compared with morphine; this is somewhat surprising considering the potency of systemic oxycodone. One explanation for this discrepancy could be that the access of oxycodone and/or some active metabolite to the central nervous system is more effective compared with morphine due to an active influx across the blood–brain barrier via an unidentified carrier protein. This carrier protein is not P-glycoprotein which is responsible for the transport of morphine and several other opioids.

The physicochemical properties of oxycodone and morphine are comparable. Both opioids are hydrophilic with a protein binding of 31–38%.

9.3 **Clinical pharmacology: pharmacokinetics**

Oxycodone is extensively metabolized with only 10% of the dose being excreted unchanged in urine. It is metabolized by the liver to oxymorphone through O-demethylation by the cytochrome P450 enzyme CYP2D6 and to noroxycodone by N-demethylation by the cytochrome P450 enzyme CYP3A4. Oxymorphone, which accounts for 10% of oxycodone metabolites, is a mu agonist with 3–5 times higher mu opioid receptor affinity than morphine. Oral oxymorphone is 10 times as potent as oral morphine based on dose and it is available as an opioid for moderate to severe pain (see Chapter 12), however, the clinical relevance of oxymorphone as an active metabolite is not as well defined as that of morphine-6-glucuronide. When the metabolism of oxycodone to oxymorphone is blocked for example, by coadministration of quinidine which blocks the CYP2D6 enzyme, the efficacy of oxycodone does not appear to be affected. The bioavailability of oxycodone is greater than 60%, which is better than that of morphine (15–60%), probably because it is protected from first-pass metabolism by its 3-methoxy substituent.

9.4 Oxycodone in renal and liver failure

The role of oxycodone in patients with renal failure is unclear. There is evidence that excretion of oxycodone, oxymorphone and noroxycodone is reduced when renal function is impaired and this has led some to comment that it is not therefore an opioid suitable for use in chronic renal failure. A case report of an female patient undergoing renal dialysis, who tolerated modified release oxycodone 50 mg twice daily with oxycodone normal release 10 mg for breakthrough pain, showed reduced concentrations of oxycodone, nor-oxycodone and oxymorphone in the post- compared to the pre-dialysis line suggesting that they were partially removed by dialysis. It is clear that further systematic observational data are required regarding its use in renal failure and until then it should be used with caution in patients with renal impairment.

The pharmacokinetics of oxycodone have been studied in end-stage liver cirrhosis before and after liver transplantation. The median elimination half-life of oxycodone was about four times longer before transplantation compared with after transplantation. The clinical relevance of this in patients with less severe liver disease is unclear.

9.5 Potential for drug interactions

Patients with pain caused by cancer are likely to be taking other medication and so the metabolism of oxycodone via the CYP2D6 and CYP3A4 systems means that it has the potential to interact with other medications being administered. A snapshot survey of 100 patients attending four adult specialist palliative care day centres revealed 24 drug combinations that were considered to represent clinically or potentially clinically important drug–drug interactions. A quarter of these combinations included analgesics, including oxycodone, so an awareness of the potential for drug interactions with oxycodone is necessary, even if their clinical relevance is unknown.

9.6 **Formulation**

The modified release formulation of oxycodone results in a bi-phasic delivery or onset of action. About 35% of the dose is rapidly released almost as if it were a normal release preparation and so provides rapid onset of analgesia. The remainder is then released over the following 6–8 h. Several studies have investigated the application of this novel delivery system and show that patients with pain achieve comparable pain relief when titrated with modified release oxycodone compared to normal release oxycodone. However, Gaertner and colleagues have postulated that this delivery system may impact upon the ability to drive while using modified release oxycodone. They investigated psychomotor function in the domains considered necessary for driving by the German regulatory authorities and attempted to prove non-inferiority of the primary end-point (patients taking modified release oxycodone would not perform statistically worse in psychomotor tests than age-matched controls). Although they concluded that stable treatment with modified release oxycodone did not preclude driving, they could not demonstrate non-inferiority. It seems the message for patients, which is similar to that for morphine, is that driving is safe on stable doses 'if you feel safe to drive'.

9.7 **Equianalagesic ratios**

Oral oxycodone is considered to be roughly twice as potent as oral morphine. However, in a randomized and controlled crossover study comparing oxycodone and morphine the equianalgesic dose ratio of oxycodone to morphine was 2:3 when oxycodone was administered first, and 3:4 when oxycodone was administered after morphine. In a prospective study investigating the factors that might predict a need to switch from oral morphine, the median morphine:oxycodone ratio in those patients who were switched from morphine to oxycodone was 1.7 but the range was large. This suggests that the ratio of 2 should be used with caution depending on the clinical situation.

9.8 **Evidence of efficacy in cancer pain**

Several randomized trials have shown comparative efficacy to both morphine and hydromorphone in patients with pain caused by cancer. A systematic review and meta-analysis of these studies showed that there was considerable heterogeneity which was explained by the control drug used. In those trials comparing oxycodone with morphine, no clinically important differences were found in efficacy. However, the authors of this review noted that the number of included studies was small and represented only 122 patients in total.

While this did not appear to compromise the statistical significance of the results it may be that larger randomized trials comparing morphine and oxycodone would help to either confirm or challenge the findings of the meta-analysis.

It can be concluded that on average morphine and oxycodone are comparable. However, significant individual differences do exist. Some of this variation in response is due to the major differences in the pharmacokinetics (metabolism and transporters) between these opioids.

9.9 Evidence of tolerability in cancer pain

Reports from two of the randomized studies suggested that oxycodone might have a superior side effect profile to morphine and subsequently reports of its improved side effects profile, and therefore tolerability, have perpetuated through the literature. In addition, the perception of an improved side effect profile has been further heightened by the practice of opioid switching. In the UK, patients will generally be commenced on morphine as first line opioid for moderate to severe pain but it is thought that approximately 10–30% of patients will not tolerate morphine. If these 10–30% of patients are then switched to oxycodone and this improves the opioid side effects experienced by the patient, it is likely that the individual clinician may perceive oxycodone to be a better tolerated opioid. In fact, in the original dose-finding prospective case series conducted by Glare and Walsh (1993), a proportion of patients required a switch from oxycodone back to morphine because of lack of effect or poorly tolerated adverse effects. The comparative tolerability of oxycodone and morphine was also assessed in the meta-analysis conducted by Reid and colleagues, and the results showed that there was no significant difference in side effect profile between oxycodone and control (morphine or hydromorphone) although significant heterogeneity did exist between the studies. Quigley also conducted a systematic review of hydromorphone in cancer pain and could not find any significant differences between hydromorphone and oxycodone.

9.10 Clinical considerations

Modified release oxycodone can be commenced at a low dose since a 5 mg tablet exists. Koizumi and colleagues (2004) investigated the safety of modified release oxycodone commenced at a low dose in 20 patients with cancer pain who were opioid naïve and reported only one withdrawal due to side effects within the 1 week study period.

9.11 **Alternative to morphine**

Reviewing the available data does not provide any evidence of oxycodone's superiority to morphine. Given its increased cost in both the UK and the USA, it is unlikely that it should replace morphine as the opioid of first choice for moderate to severe cancer pain. The Scottish Medicines Consortium (www.scottishmedicines consortium.org.uk) has recommended modified release oxycodone for patients in whom modified release morphine is ineffective or not tolerated, endorsing the position of morphine as first choice opioid. However, the available data also confirm that oxycodone is an equivalent alternative to morphine and therefore represents an important drug for use in pain caused by cancer.

Key References

Barakzoy, A.S. and Moss, A.H. (2006). Efficacy of the World Health Organization analgesic ladder to treat pain in end-stage renal disease. *J. Am. Soc. Nephrol.*, **17**, 3198–3203.

Beaver, W., Wallenstein, S.L., Rogers, A. and Houde, R.W. (1978). Analgesic studies of codeine and oxycodone in patients with cancer. II. Comparisons of intramuscular oxycodone with intramuscular morphine and codeine. *J. Pharmacol. Exp. Ther.*, **207**, 101–8.

Bruera, E., Belzile, M., Pituskin, E., Fainsinger, R., Darke, A., Harsanyi, Z., et al. (1998). Randomized, double-blind, cross-over trial comparing safety and efficacy of oral controlled-release oxycodone with controlled-release morphine in patients with cancer pain. *J. Clin. Oncol.*, **16**, 3222–9.

Glare, P.A. and Walsh, D.T. (1993). Dose-ranging study of oxycodone for chronic pain in advanced cancer. *J. Clin. Oncol.*, **11**, 973–8.

Hanks, G.W. and Reid, C. (2005). Contribution to variability in response to opioids. *Support. Care Cancer*, **13**, 145–52.

Heiskanen, T. and Kalso, E. (1997). Controlled-release oxycodone and morphine in cancer related pain, *Pain*, **73**, 37–45.

Kalso, E. and Vainio, A. (1990). Morphine and oxycodone hydrochloride in the management of cancer pain. *Clin. Pharmacol. Ther.*, **47,** 639–46.

Kalso, E., Vainio, A., Mattila, M.J., Rosenberg, P.H. and Seppala, T. (1990). Morphine and oxycodone in the management of cancer pain: plasma levels determined by chemical and radioreceptor assays. *Pharmacol. Toxicol.*, **67**, 322–8.

Kaplan, R., Parris, W.C-V., Citron, M.L., Zhukovsky, D., Reder, R.F., Buckley, B.J., et al. (1998). Comparison of controlled-release and immediate-release oxycodone tablets in patients with cancer pain. *J. Clin. Oncol.*, **16**, 3230–7.

Klepstad, P., Kaasa, S., Cherny, N., Hanks, G. and De Conno, F. (2005). Pain and pain treatments in European palliative care units. A cross sectional survey from the European Association for Palliative Care Research Network. *Palliat. Med.,* **19**, 477–84.

Koizumi, W., Toma, H., Watanabe, K., Katamaya, K., Kawahara, M., Matsui, K., *et al.* (2004). Efficacy and tolerability of cancer pain management with controlled-release oxycodone tablets in opioid-naive cancer pain patients, starting with 5 mg tablets. *Jpn. J. Clin. Oncol.,* **34**, 608–14.

Lee, M.A., Leng, M.E.F., and Cooper, R. (2005). Measurements of plasma oxycodone, noroxycodone and oxymorphone levels in a patient with bilateral nephrectomy who is undergoing heamodialysis. *Palliat. Med.,* **19**, 259–60.

Mandema, J.W., Kaiko, R.F., Oshlack, B., Reder, R.F. and Stanski, D.R. (1996). Characterization and validation of a pharmacokinetic model for controlled-release oxycodone. *Br. J.Clin. Pharmacol.,* **42**, 747–56.

Mucci-LoRusso, P., Berman, B.S., Silberstein, P.T., Citron, M.L., Bressler, L., Weinstein, S.M., *et al.* (1998). Controlled-release oxycodone with controlled-release morphine in the treatment of cancer pain: a randomized, double-blind, parallel-group study. *Eur. J. Pain,* **2**, 239–49.

Quigley, C. (2004). Opioid switching to improve pain relief and drug tolerability. *Cochrane Database Syst. Rev.,* **3**, CD004847.

Reid, C.M., Martin, R.M., Sterne, J.A.C., Davies, A.N. and Hanks, G.W. (2006). Oxycodone for cancer-related pain. Meta-analysis of randomized controlled trials. *Arch. Intern. Med.,* **166**, 837–43.

Ross, J.R., Riley, J., Quigley, C. and Welsh, K.I. (2006). Clinical pharmacology and pharmacotherapy of opioid switching in cancer patients. *Oncologist,* **11**, 765–73.

Wilcock, A., Thomas, J., Frisby, J., Webster, M., Keeley, V., Finn, G., *et al.* (2005). Potential for drug interactions involving cytochrome P450 in patients attending palliative day care centres: a multicentre audit. *Br. J. Clin. Pharm.,* **60**, 326–29.

Chapter 10

Hydromorphone

Naeem Ahmed and Catherine E. Urch

> ### Key points
> - Hydromorphone is a potent opioid analgesic.
> - It has an analgesic and side effect profile similar to morphine.
> - It is an alternative to morphine in patients with moderate to severe cancer pain with inadequate analgesia or unacceptable side effects due to morphine.

10.1 Background

Hydromorphone is a semi-synthetic opioid which was synthesised by Knoll in Germany in the 1920s. It was introduced into clinical practice in 1926. Hydromorphone has been used in North America for many years but was introduced in the UK only in 1997 for moderate to severe cancer pain. In the UK it is being used increasingly in this context, however, in North America it has also been used extensively for postoperative pain. In spite of its widespread use over many years there is still doubt over its potency in relation to morphine, which has been reported variably as morphine: hydromorphone 4:1–8:1. In July 2005 the modified release preparation was withdrawn from the American market after fears of toxicity and fatally high plasma levels when taken with alcohol.

10.2 Pharmacokinetics

Hydromorphone is a hydrogenated ketone analogue of morphine and is structurally very similar to morphine. Its chemical name is 4,5 alpha-epoxy-3-hydroxy-17-methyl morphinan-6-one. It is believed to mimic the effects of endogenous opioids and, like morphine, it acts primarily on the mu opioid receptor and to a lesser degree on delta receptors. It has no effect on kappa receptors.

10.2.1 Oral administration

Hydromorphone is absorbed from the upper small intestine following oral administration. It is extensively metabolized by the liver.

Approximately 62% of an oral dose is eliminated by the liver on first pass resulting in a bioavailability in the range of 12–50% depending on interindividual variation. The onset of analgesia is at approximately 30 min with a duration of action of approximately 4 h following administration of the normal release preparation. For modified release preparations, the bioavailability is similar to the normal release preparation, however, the time to peak plasma levels is 3–4 times longer (i.e. 1.3–2 h) with a duration of action of either 12 or 24 h depending upon the preparation.

10.2.2 **Parenteral administration**

The onset of action after intravenous adminstration of hydromorphone is approximately 5 min although maximum effect is not achieved for up to 20 min. Hydromorphone is 10 times more lipid soluble than morphine and therefore its onset of action is faster than morphine but slower than that of more lipid soluble drugs such as fentanyl. Bioavailability following subcutaneous administration is 78%. Parenteral formulations are not currently available in the UK.

10.2.3 **Rectal administration**

Studies of rectal absorption produce conflicting results, but in practice the rectal route appears comparable to the oral route. Rectal formulations are not currently available in the UK.

10.2.4 **Intranasal administration**

A hydromorphone hydrochloride nasal spray is being developed currently and clinical trials show rapid absorption and bioavailability higher than oral doses. This route avoids gastrointestinal degradation and hepatic first pass metabolism.

10.2.5 **Spinal administration**

Hydromorphone given by the epidural route may be absorbed into the local tissues, traverse the dura and gain access to the cerebrospinal fluid or be absorbed into the systemic circulation. The concentration of hydromorphone in the cerebrospinal fluid at the cervical level peaks 1 h after lumbar epidural administration. The epidural to parenteral equianalgesic ratio is 1:2. The duration of action following a single epidural dose is very variable and has been reported as between 7.7 and 19.3 h. Epidural formulations are not currently available in the UK.

10.2.6 **Hydromorphone metabolism**

Hydromorphone is extensively metabolized in the liver. The main metabolite is hydromorphone-3-glucuronide (H3G), which does not have any analgesic properties. Two minor metabolites, dihydroisomorphine and dihydromorphine, are pharmacologically active and are metabolized to 6-glucuronides. Unconjugated hydromorphone is also excreted. Unlike morphine, hydromorphone does not have a 6-glucuronide metabolite.

Only a small amount of hydromorphone is excreted in the urine unchanged, most of the drug is excreted as hydromorphone-3-glucuronide. The elimination half-life after an intravenous dose is about 2.3 h.

10.3 **Hydromorphone in renal and hepatic disease**

In renal failure, hydromorphone and its metabolites accumulate resulting in opioid toxicity. The mean ratio of H3G to hydromorphone may increase to 100:1. H3G is 2.5 times as potent as M3G as a neuroexcitant. Myoclonus, allodynia and seizures have been reported in patients with high levels of H3G. As for all other renally excreted opioids, a report of increased pain in the context of confusion, myoclonus or other features of opioid toxicity should prompt the physician to check the patient's renal function and consider switching to an alternative opioid. In liver disease, where the hepatic blood flow or metabolic function is altered, hydromorphone bioavailability will vary. This may be of clinical importance in congestive heart failure, hepatic cirrhosis, circulatory collapse and shock.

10.4 **Equianalgesic ratios**

There is some debate over equianalgesic conversion tables, particularly for hydromorphone. In the UK, the manufacturer suggests that oral hydromorphone is 7.5 times as potent as oral morphine, hence capsule sizes of 1.3 and 2.6 mg. Equianalgesic tables are often derived from single dose studies producing slightly different results than are obtained with repeated dosing. Unlike other opioids, potency ratios for hydromorphone are not bidirectional. An equianalgesic ratio of 7.1 is quoted when switching from morphine to hydromorphone but ratios of 4:1–8:1 are reported when switching in the other direction. The reported oral equianalgesic ratio for morphine to hydromorphone is 7.5:1 and the parenteral equianalgesic ratio is 7:1, so when converting from oral to subcutaneous hydromorphone, the dose should be divided by two, presuming an oral to parenteral potency ratio for morphine of 1:2.

10.5 **Administration and formulation**

Hydromorphone can be administered by several different routes: oral, rectal, subcutaneous, intravenous and spinally. Less commonly, it may be given intranasally. A transdermal preparation will also be available in the near future.

In the UK hydromorphone is available as normal release Palladone® capsules, 1.3 and 2.6 mg, modified release Palladone® SR capsules, 2, 4, 8, 16 and 24 mg. In North America it is available in normal release formulations marketed as Dilaudid® tablets or oral liquid, parenteral formulations and as a 3 mg suppository. As for morphine, normal release preparations are given 4-hourly, and modified release preparations 12-hourly.

10.6 **Evidence of efficacy and tolerability**

Hydromorphone has similar side effects to morphine. Some studies suggest that hydromorphone may cause less pruritis, sedation, nausea and vomiting than morphine but other studies fail to show such a difference. Quigley (2002) conducted a systematic review of hydromorphone in cancer pain and could not find any significant differences between hydromorphone and oxycodone. As for all strong opioids tolerance to some side effects may develop with repeated administration.

10.7 **Alternative to morphine**

As documented in previous chapters, oral morphine is the drug of choice for chronic pain due to cancer, however, a significant proportion of patients do not achieve adequate pain relief with morphine, usually because of unmanageable side effects. Hydromorphone has a role as an alternative to morphine in patients who require an opioid switch.

Key references

Altea Therapeutics (2007). Altea Therapeutics completes phase 2 clinical study in acute pain for its hydromorphone transdermal patch. http://www.alteatherapeutics.com/ accessed 2 April 2007.

Anderson, R., Saiers, J.H., Abram, S. and Schlicht, C. (2001). Accuracy in equianalgesic dosing: conversion dilemmas. *J. Pain Symptom Manage.*, **21**, 397–406.

Murray, A. and Hagen, N.A. (2005). Hydromorphone. *J. Pain Symptom Manage.*, **29**(S5), 57–66.

Quigley, C. (2002). Hydromorphone for acute and chronic pain. *Cochrane Database Syst. Rev.*,**1**, CD00347.

Quigley, C. and Wiffen, P. (2003). A systematic review of hydromorphone in acute and chronic pain, *J. Pain Symptom Manage.*, **25**, 169–78.

Sarhill, N., Walsh, D. and Nelson, K.A. (2001). Hydromorphone: pharmacology and clinical applications in cancer patients. *Support. Care Cancer*, **9**, 84–96.

Chapter 11

Methadone

Matthew Makin

> **Key points**
> - Methadone is a potent opioid analgesic with other non opioid properties.
> - It has an analgesic and side effect profile similar to morphine.
> - It is difficult to use because of a long and variable half-life.
> - Conversion to methadone from other opioids is complex so it is best used in specialist settings

11.1 Background

In many of the discussion forums on pain management and palliative medicine, methadone is suggested as the answer to a variety of 'challenging' pain syndromes. Methadone can be a useful alternative to other strong opioids, but its use should not be considered lightly.

Methadone is a synthetic strong opioid analgesic. It was originally developed as a battlefield analgesic in the 1940s. It is cheap and is the only long-acting opioid that can be given as a liquid. It is best known in the UK for the treatment of opioid dependence. The use of methadone in the treatment of pain was, until recently, limited to a few individuals working from specialist centres, however, over the past decade anecdotal reports and a number of open case series and clinical trials have described the successful use of methadone, principally in cancer pain syndromes that have responded poorly to high doses of other strong opioids.

11.2 Pharmacology and pharmacokinetics

The analgesic action of methadone is mediated via opioid receptors in the central nervous system; it has strong affinity for mu, with less, but still appreciable affinity for delta and very weak affinity for kappa receptors. The high affinity for the mu receptor is matched by high efficacy at this receptor. Methadone also has a broad spectrum of other receptor affinities; of particular interest are its re-uptake inhibitory properties towards N-methyl-D-aspartate (NMDA) receptor antagonist, serotonin and noradrenaline. There is also some evidence to suggest that it may directly interact with neuronal voltage-dependent sodium channels in a manner similar to local anaesthetics. It has been suggested that these opioid and additional non-opioid properties may be of clinical relevance, particularly in the management of neuropathic pain. The putative advantages of methadone in relation to its activity at the NMDA receptor are controversial, however. Methadone has been shown to interact with the NMDA receptor *in vitro*, but electrophysiological and *in vivo* studies have not established conclusively that it acts as a 'functional' NMDA receptor antagonist.

Methadone is highly lipophilic and is rapidly and effectively absorbed when given via the oral route and rectally. It has a high oral bio-availability of 80% with a range of 41–99%, although there is some metabolism in the wall of the gut by the cytochrome system CYP3A4. Methadone is highly bound to the protein alpha-1-acid-glycoprotein and undergoes considerable tissue distribution; it is this peripheral reservoir that sustains plasma levels during chronic treatment. Studies of patients using methadone in the context of chemical dependency have calculated high volumes of distribution indicating that during chronic treatment only approximately 1% of the drug is present in the blood.

There have been few studies to characterize the kinetics of methadone in humans. One study suggested that the terminal elimination half-life of methadone was long (33–46 h) and possibly longer in those with chemical dependency. Methadone crosses the placenta and is measurable in the breast milk of those using the drug. Measuring plasma concentrations after oral dosing cannot be used for predicting and adjusting dosage in patients on long-term methadone therapy.

11.3 Potential for drug interactions

Elimination of methadone is mediated by hepatic oxidative biotransformation, and renal N-demethylation. Methadone's N-demethylation is mediated via the cytochrome P450 group. The main enzyme mediating the N-demethylation of methadone is CYP3A4 with lesser involvement of CYP1A2 and CYP2D6, and hence drug interactions are related to inducers or inhibitors of this cytochrome system (see Table 11.1). Genetic polymorphisms of these cytochrome systems exist that can result in extremes of poor or rapid metabolism; this may account for the large interindividual variations in methadone pharmacology. There are also risks of other side effects: the co-administration of benzodiazepines can potentiate sedation and respiratory depression, and the co-administration of risperidone may precipitate an opioid withdrawal reaction.

Table 11.1 Common drug interactions	
3A4 inducers	**3A4 inhibitors**
Reduce effect of methadone	Increase effect of methadone
Anticonvulsants	Antidepressants
Corticosteroids	Antiretrovirals
Antitubercular drugs	Antifungals
	Antipsychotics

11.4 **Methadone in renal failure**

Methadone does not accumulate in renal failure nor does it cross renal dialysis membranes, rather the majority (approximately 70%) is excreted via the gut. These properties suggest advantages over other strong opioids in patients with renal impairment or on dialysis because of end-stage renal failure.

11.5 **Administration and formulation**

Methadone can be given by mouth as a liquid or tablet, or injected intramuscularly or subcutaneously. In clinical practice it is used as a racemic mixture of (levorotatory) L-methadone and (dextrorotatory) D-methadone. It is produced as a hydrochloride salt in a solution having a pH range of 3–6. In the UK racemic methadone is available in 5 mg tablets as well as solutions of varying strengths (1 mg/1 mL, 10 mg/1 mL and 20 mg/1 mL), and a range of strengths of ampoule for injection can be obtained. In the USA racemic methadone tablets 5–10 mg and a dispersible 40 mg tablet can be prescribed along with a range of oral solutions and preparations for injection. The analgesic action of the racemic presentation is almost entirely attributable to the L-methadone content which is many times more potent than the D-isomer. D-methadone does not cause respiratory depression but does behave as a cough suppressant.

Methadone is also well absorbed when given as a suppository and its long half-life means a relatively long dose interval. The pharmacokinetics of rectal methadone is very similar to oral methadone with a rapid absorption, extensive distribution and a slow elimination phase. There are a number of clinical reports of its effective use per rectum, with proctitis reported only as a rare complication. The use of continuous subcutaneous infusion (CSCI) of methadone has been discouraged in the past, but the addition of dexamethasone to the infusion and the use of dilute solutions of methadone with frequent infusion site changes have allowed methadone to be administered subcutaneously. The successful use of intravenous infusions of low dose methadone has also been described in small case series. There would appear little advantage in giving methadone spinally, owing to its rapid absorption and plasma accumulation via other routes, but epidural use has been reported.

11.6 **Evidence of efficacy**

There have been many case reports of the successful use of methadone in cancer pain as well as an increasing number of retrospective and prospective open case studies. The primary indication for considering methadone as an alternative strong opioid is when a patient with a challenging pain syndrome develops resistant dose limiting side effects to morphine or other strong opioids, usually with relatively high doses, for example, mean equivalent daily dose of morphine (MEDD) >200 mg. These side effects will often prohibit escalation of the previous opioid dose and give rise to inadequate analgesia, despite the use of co-analgesics and/or techniques appropriate to the pain syndrome. In such circumstances, it has been suggested that methadone may have specific advantages as an alternative strong opioid because of the synergistic actions of its opioid and non-opioid effects, lack of active metabolites, and the unidirectional cross-tolerance it displays with other mu opioid agonists. In a double-blind randomized and controlled trial, methadone showed an analgesic advantage over placebo in patients with treatment resistant neuropathic pain, and has demonstrated analgesic activity in other neuropathic pain syndromes.

Other than cost, there are no advantages of using methadone as a first line strong opioid, even in neuropathic pain, and this has been confirmed in clinical trials. In a randomized double-blind study Bruera and colleagues (2004) compared morphine and methadone as the first line strong opioid in the management of cancer pain in 103 patients. The authors concluded that methadone produced similar levels of analgesia compared with morphine but were unable to show whether methadone had any specific advantages in those few patients identified as having cancer-related neuropathic pain as the numbers were small. This study concurred with three other studies directly comparing morphine with methadone, which reported that similar pain relief was achieved with both drugs.

The unidirectional cross-tolerance seen in animal and clinical studies between methadone and other strong opioids infers that if methadone is to be used, it is best used as a second or third line strong opioid. This is because although there are a number of effective guidelines for conversion from other strong opioids to methadone, there are no such recommendations on how to convert from methadone to other strong opioids, if this were necessary.

11.7 **Evidence of tolerability**

Methadone shares numerous side effects common to the strong opioid analgesics, such as constipation, nausea, vomiting, dizziness, drowsiness and pruritus. Studies comparing oral and parenteral morphine and methadone have failed to show any significant differences in efficacy or adverse effects.

Patients usually require short dosing intervals to achieve adequate pain relief initially, with longer dosing intervals for maintenance of analgesia. Significant toxicity, notably drowsiness, coma and respiratory depression, has been reported when methadone dose has been increased too frequently, conversion doses were too high, or dosing intervals too close. This can occur as a result of the long and unpredictable half-life of methadone, and it is the risk of accumulation leading to toxicity that has encouraged many authors to recommend an initial dose titration phase when converting from any other strong opioid to methadone. Prolongation of the QT interval and the development of life-threatening torsade de pointes ventricular tachycardia have also been reported in association with methadone use.

11.8 **Strategies for conversion to methadone**

The best strategy for switching from any opioid to methadone is yet to be determined; there have been no studies thus far comparing the relative efficacy or safety of different guidelines. Conversion strategies can be divided into two main approaches; 'by-the-clock' and 'ad libitum'. (See Table 11.2.)

11.8.1 **Methadone by-the-clock**

The Edmonton regimen involves an approach overlapping methadone with the previous opioid over 3 days. On the first day, the previous opioid dose is reduced by 30–50% and methadone is given every 8 h using a morphine to methadone ratio of 10:1. On the second day, the dose of the original opioid is reduced by a further 30–50% and the methadone dose is increased if pain control is poor. On the third day, the previous opioid is discontinued and methadone is given every 8 h with a rescue dose of methadone, calculated as 10% of the daily methadone dose, given as required. This approach was used in a prospective study of 108 cancer patients; conversion to methadone was completed in 103 patients with significant improvements in pain control leading the authors to conclude that this was a safe and effective strategy.

Mercadante reports a strategy of rapid conversion from the previous opioid to methadone. This involves stopping the previous opioid and immediately substituting methadone, using a morphine to

Table 11.2 Examples of dose conversion regimens	
UK model for switching from morphine to methadone (ad libitum) from Morley and Makin (1998)	Edmonton model for switching from morphine to methadone (by-the-clock) from Bruera *et al.* (1996)
• Previous opioid stopped and replaced by fixed dose of methadone given PRN • Patient on <300 mg of morphine/24 h– morphine:methadone = 10:1 • Patient on >300 mg of morphine/24 h– fixed dose of 30 mg methadone • Methadone given PRN not more than 3- hourly • Day 6: amount of methadone administered over previous 2 days noted, and converted to a 12-hourly regimen • Methadone requirements expected to decrease during days 2 and 3 and reach steady state on days 4 and 5	• Day 1: decrease morphine dose by 30% and replace with po methadone 8-hourly— morphine:methadone = 10:1 • Day 2: decrease morphine by another 30%. Methadone dose increased if patient experiences moderate to severe pain. Transient pain treated with short-acting opioids • Day 3: discontinue morphine. Maintain patient on 8-hourly methadone plus 10% of daily methadone dose administered as rescue dose for breakthrough pain
Data sourced from Brown *et al.* (2004)	

methadone ratio of 4:1 for patients receiving <90 mg of morphine/ day, a ratio of 8:1 for patients receiving 90–300 mg of morphine/day and a ratio of 12:1 for patients receiving >300 mg of morphine per day. Methadone is given at the calculated dose as a liquid every 8 h with three extra 'rescue doses' allowed each day. These rescue doses are calculated as one-sixth of the daily methadone dose. The day-to-day methadone dose is then titrated depending upon the requirements of rescue doses.

11.8.2 Methadone ad libitum

The emphasis of an ad libitum approach is the avoidance of toxicity during the initial dose titration phase due to methadone accumulation. It relies on stopping the previous opioid and the prescription of a 'fixed' dose of methadone, with the patient determining the dose interval, as long as this is not more than 3-hourly. A morphine to methadone ratio of 10:1 is advised, with a ceiling dose imposed for dose titration. The regimen that is now accepted most commonly, in the UK, recommends a fixed dose of methadone at one-tenth of the 24 h equivalent oral morphine dose (EOMD), with a ceiling dose of 30 mg for titration when the EOMD exceeds 300 mg/24 h. This regimen advocates conversion to twice daily methadone on the sixth day of dose titration. The ceiling dose of 30 mg was decided upon after Morley and Makin (1998) examined reports of 146 successful conversions to methadone from 32 different UK hospices.

There have been a number of variations to the Morley–Makin approach, and lower ceiling doses have been suggested. A recent prospective study in a Chinese population used a morphine to methadone ratio of 12:1 with a ceiling dose of 30 mg of methadone. This ad libitum regimen was continued until the demand for methadone was stabilized. Other ad libitum approaches have advocated even higher morphine to methadone dose ratios.

11.9 **Alternative to morphine**

There is no evidence that methadone is superior to morphine as an analgesic. It is not easy to use, and can be hazardous because of its pharmacology; it is best initiated therefore as an alternative opioid in a specialist inpatient setting by a team experienced in its use. It is, however, cheap and anecdotal experience suggests it may be useful in challenging pain syndromes where patients have failed to tolerate adequate doses of alternative opioids.

Key references

Brown, R., Kraus, C., Fleming, M. and Reddy, S. (2004). Methadone: applied pharmacology and use as adjunctive treatment in chronic pain. *Postgrad. Med. J.*, **80**, 654–9.

Bruera, E., Palmer, J.L., Bosnjak, S., Rico, M.A., Moyano, J., Sweeney, C., et al. (2004). Methadone versus morphine as a first-line strong opioid for cancer pain: a randomized, double-blind study, *J. Clin. Oncol.*, **22**, 185–92.

Fishbain, D.A., Cutler, R.B., Cole, B., Lewis, J., Rosomoff, R.S. and Rosomoff, H.L. (2003). Medico-legal rounds: medico-legal issues and alleged breaches of 'standards of medical care' in opioid rotation to methadone: a case report. *Pain Med.*, **4**, 195–201.

Morley, J.S. and Makin, M.K. (1998). The use of methadone in cancer pains poorly responsive to other opioids. *Pain Rev.*, **5**, 51–8.

Morley, J.S., Bridson, J., Nash, T.P., Miles, J.B., White, S. and Makin, M.K. (2004). Low-dose methadone has an analgesic effect in neuropathic pain: a double-blind randomized controlled crossover trial. *Palliat. Med.*, **17**, 576–87.

Nicholson, A.B. (2004). Methadone for cancer pain. *Cochrane Database Syst. Rev.* (2), CD003971.

Chapter 12

Other alternative oral opioids

Matthew Makin

> ### Key points
> - Some opioids may have advantages over morphine in specific circumstances because of their pharmacokinetic and pharmacodynamic profiles.
> - The fentanyl analogues may have greatest utility for episodic pain.
> - Theoretical advantages such as NMDA receptor antagonism and inhibition of the re-uptake of biogenic monoamines have not been confirmed as producing better efficacy or tolerability in clinical studies.

12.1 Background

The mu opioid agonist morphine remains the oral opioid of first choice for chronic cancer pain.

There are circumstances, however, when clinicians encounter patients already using other oral strong opioids, or need to consider their use. This may be prompted by a patient's intolerance of the alternative oral strong opioids we have discussed already in this book, or by a desire to take advantage of the different pharmacokinetic or pharmacodynamic profiles that other strong opioids may offer. This may be the case when the use of a rapid onset, short-acting drug is required, for example, for breakthrough pain, or in cases of hepatic or renal impairment.

12.2 Potential advantages of some opioids

Many of the commonly used strong opioids are metabolized through the liver microsomal cytochrome P450(CYP) system. CYP2D6 and CYP3A4 are responsible for the metabolism of many opioids. They are involved in the metabolism of a wide range of other drugs and are susceptible to the influence of drugs that are enzyme inhibitors or inducers, liver disease, or genetic variation. Opioids such as oxymorphone may have particular utility in such circumstances as its metabolism is not dependent on CYP2D6 and 3A4. It has also been suggested that some strong opioids may have advantages over others because they possess a broader spectrum of action, such as the ability to block the re-uptake of biogenic monoamines or to act as functional antagonists at the N-methyl-D-aspartate (NMDA) receptor (e.g. levorphanol or tramadol). Some authors propose that opioids acting as partial agonists (e.g. buprenorphine, pentazocine and butorphanol) may be useful in the management of cancer pain characterized by hyperalgesia. These hypotheses, though credible, have yet to be proven in large-scale clinical trials. Research is also underway into whether oral kappa opioid agonists that have minimal penetration into the central nervous system (CNS), and opioids that have mixed agonism at the mu and delta opioid receptors provide a better balance between analgesia and side effects such as dysphoria, sedation and respiratory depression than other opioids.

The following section is divided into alternative strong opioids that may have significant utility in the future for chronic pain management (oxymorphone and levorphanol), short-acting opioids that may have potential in the management of breakthrough pain (sufentanil, remifentanil), opioids that have been discontinued or proven unhelpful (Morphidex®, dipipanone, phenazocine and dextromoramide), and drugs that should be avoided in cancer pain management (pethidine, butorphanol, nalbuphine and pentazocine).

12.3 **Potentially useful alternative strong opioids**

12.3.1 **Oxymorphone (Opana and Opana ER®)**

Oxymorphone is an active metabolite of oxycodone. It has been marketed as a strong opioid analgesic since 1959. Oxymorphone is about three times as potent as morphine with a similar onset of action (30 min) and an elimination half-life of between 7 and 9 h. In the past it was administered most commonly by suppository; it is now available in the USA as normal release (Opana®) and modified release (Opana ER®) oral preparations. Opana ER® can be administered at 12-hourly intervals. With a predictable dose–response and pharmacokinetics that have been shown to be linear and dose proportional (unlike methadone and levorphanol), oxymorphone promises to be a useful alternative strong opioid in chronic cancer pain management. It may be particularly useful for patients prone to drug–drug interactions since it is not metabolized through CYP3A4 or CYP2D6. Oxymorphone is not currently available in the UK.

12.3.2 **Levorphanol**

Levorphanol (levo-3-hydroxy-N-methylmorphinan) is a synthetic strong opioid that is the only available opioid agonist of the morphinan series. It shares a number of pharmacological properties with methadone. Like methadone, it displays unidirectional cross-tolerance to other opioids and has a broad spectrum of action at mu, delta and kappa opioid receptors. It has been shown to bind in a non-competitive manner at the channel blocking site at the NMDA receptor; it also inhibits the re-uptake of biogenic monoamines such as serotonin and noradrenaline *in vitro*.

Like morphine, levorphanol undergoes glucuronidation in the liver, and the glucuronidated products are excreted in the urine. The efficacy and acceptability of levorphanol have been subjected to a well-designed dose–response clinical trial. In this study, levorphanol was shown to have an analgesic effect at low and high doses (approximately 3 and 10 mg/day) in neuropathic pain. The investigators concluded that reduction in the intensity of pain was significantly greater during treatment with higher doses of opioid, however, these doses produced more side effects without significant additional benefit in terms of other outcomes such as affective distress, functioning and sleep (Table 12.1). Levorphanol is not currently available in the UK.

Table 12.1 Equianalgesic dose table*				
Opioid analgesic	Equianalgesic doses (mg)	Half-life (hours)	Peak effect (hours)	Duration (hours)
Morphine	10 mg SC	2–3	0.5–1	3–4
	20–30 mg PO	2–3	1–2	3–6
Oxymorphone	1 mg SC	1–2	0.5–1	3–6
	10 mg PR	1–2	1.5–3	4–6
	15 mg PO			
Levorphanol*	4 mg PO	12–15	1–2	3–6

* Note this table is a guide and should be used with caution. The phenomenon of incomplete cross-tolerance may necessitate a relative dose reduction and care should be used in converting to levorphanol because, like methadone, it has a short duration of action but a long half-life which can lead to accumulation and toxicity with regular dose intervals.

12.3.3 **Analogues of fentanyl**

The synthetic analogues of fentanyl are playing an increasing role in the management of breakthrough pain. Fentanyl and alfentanil have also been used as continuous subcutaneous infusions in cases of morphine intolerance, particularly in patients with renal impairment. Other synthetic analogues have been considered as self-administered short-acting opioids for various types of breakthrough pain. Sufentanil, for example, has been used off-licence both intranasally and via a delivery device similar to an insulin pen. Sufentanil is approximately 5–10 times as potent as fentanyl and can be used as a lower volume alternative to fentanyl in syringe drivers. Remifentanil is a very short-acting opioid with a half-life of between 1 and 20 min; it is usually used in anaesthesia. It is metabolized peripherally rather than by the liver, and so accumulation does not occur in cases of hepatic failure. Remifentanil is approximately 2100 times more potent than morphine and 70 times more potent than alfentanil. Sufentanil is not currently available in the UK.

12.4 **Drugs with little or no proven efficacy or which have been withdrawn**

12.4.1 **Dextromethorphan and morphine (Morphidex®)**

Dextromethorphan is a salt of the methyl ether dextrorotatory isomer of levorphanol and, although structurally similar, should not strictly be classified as an opioid because it has little or no affinity for opioid receptors although, like levorphanol, it has affinity for the non-competitive binding site at the NMDA receptor. It has been used extensively as a cough suppressant, however, interest was generated by preclinical and clinical studies suggesting potential in the addition of NMDA receptor antagonists, such as dextromethorphan, to opioid analgesics such as morphine. The theory was that dextromethorphan would potentiate the analgesic effect of morphine, reducing analgesic tolerance and improving the dose response in neuropathic pain syndromes. In practice this proved not to be the case, indeed no statistically significant differences between treatment groups in any primary or secondary efficacy variables were demonstrated in a well-designed multicentre trial comparing morphine with morphine plus dextromethorphan (Morphidex®). It is not currently available in the UK.

12.4.2 **Dipipanone**

Dipipanone is structurally similar to methadone and dextromoramide, and is combined with cyclizine under the trade name Diconal® (dipipanone 10 mg with cyclizine 30 mg) in the UK. Although some patients preferred Diconal® to other strong opioids, the combination of drugs in this preparation limited dose escalation and hence wider utility in chronic cancer pain.

12.4.3 **Phenazocine**

Phenazocine acts rapidly when given sublingually, and with an onset of analgesic action in some cases of less than 30 min, it was favoured in the management of breakthrough pain. One 5 mg tablet was roughly equivalent to 25 mg of morphine. It had a rather unique mode of administration in some units; it fitted neatly into the centre of a Polo Mint® to mask its bitter taste. It is no longer available in the UK.

12.4.4 **Dextromoramide (Palfium®)**

Dextromoramide is another strong opioid with a rapid onset of action which was discontinued in 2003. Its duration of analgesic action is shorter than morphine and has been observed to reduce to 1–2 h with repeated administration and development of analgesic tolerance.

12.4.5 **Pethidine**

Pethidine, once a very popular opioid in the treatment of acute and chronic pain, has recently, and with good reason, fallen from grace. Some surgical teams favour its use in biliary and renal colic due to its putative antispasmodic properties, however, there is no evidence from pragmatic clinical trials that pethidine is any better than morphine in such cases. Pethidine has significant disadvantages when used in the treatment of chronic pain, because of its short half-life and duration of analgesic action (approximately 2–3 h). When given in repeated doses, plasma levels of the metabolite norpethidine, which has a longer elimination half-life than pethidine, can increase, particularly in association with renal impairment. Accumulation of norpethidine can lead to neurotoxicity that is not reversed by naloxone. Symptoms include myoclonus, hallucinations, delirium and convulsions. In patients concomitantly taking other drugs that inhibit the re-uptake of serotonin an unpleasant serotonin syndrome can also develop.

12.4.6 **Butorphanol, nalbuphine and pentazocine**

These opioids are mixed agonist–antagonist drugs producing agonist effects at one, usually the mu, receptor and antagonist effects at other opioid receptors. Their utility is limited, and they are probably best avoided for cancer pain as they are reported as having more psychotomimetic side effects than pure agonists, they have an analgesic ceiling, and they have the potential to promote acute withdrawal effects in patients who have developed physical dependence on other strong opioids. Butorphanol and nalbuphine are not currently available in the UK.

Key references

Barnett, M. (2001). Alternative opioids to morphine in palliative care: a review of current practice and evidence. *Postgrad. Med. J.,* **77**, 371–378.

Urch, C.E., Carr, S. and Minton, O. (2004). A retrospective review of the use of alfentanil in a hospital palliative care setting. *Palliat. Med.,* **18**, 516–9.

Fine, P. and Portenoy, R.K. *Opioid analgesia* (2004). McGraw Hill, New York.

Sloan, P., Slatkin, N. and Ahdieh, H. (2005). Effectiveness and safety of oral extende-release oxymorphone for the treatment of cancer pain: a pilot study. *Support Care Cancer*, **13**, 57–65.

Dale, O., Hjortkjaer, R. and Kharasch, E.D. (2002) Nasal administration of opioids for pain management in adults. *Acta Anaesthesiol Scand.*, **46**, 759–70.

Part V

Alternative routes of administration

Chapter 13

Transdermal opioids

Luke Feathers and Christina Faull

> **Key points**
> Transdermal opioids
> - Can provide good pain relief.
> - Are useful when the oral route of administration is not possible.
> - Should not be used when rapid titration of analgesia is required.
> - May aid compliance.
> - May cause less constipation and somnolence than morphine.
> - May be the patient's method of choice.

13.1 Introduction

Delivery of drugs transdermally has been possible for many years. The basic technology is that low molecular weight lipophilic molecules, contained in a drug reservoir, migrate across the skin into the capillary blood stream because of a concentration gradient. The two self-adhesive opioid patches, fentanyl (1995) and buprenorphine (2002) have sophisticated pharmaceutical technologies that ensure predictable and constant dose delivery.

13.2 Practical considerations for transdermal opioid use

The patch strength to be used should be calculated from manufacturer's guidelines or other guidance, as discussed below. The patch should be applied and oral medication continued for the next 12 h, for example, the last dose of 12-hourly opioid is given as the patch is applied, or three further doses of 4-hourly opioid are required. Patients require an appropriate analgesic for breakthrough pain and patients should be warned that they may experience more breakthrough pain than usual in the first 1–3 days.

13.2.1 **Advice to patients**

- Patches should be stuck to a flat, clean, dry area of hairless skin, usually on the trunk or back or on the upper outer arm. Men may need to cut, not shave, body hair, as the skin integrity must be preserved.
- The transdermal patch should be pressed firmly in place with the palm of the hand for approximately 30 s. If the edges of the patch begin to peel off, the edges may be taped down with suitable skin tape.
- Patients are able to shower and swim with the patches in place.
- Hot baths and directly applied heat will rapidly increase absorption, as will raised body temperature from pyrexia.
- If a patch falls off, a new one should be applied.
- Used patches should be folded sticky side together, and disposed of safely or returned to a pharmacist.

The dose of the patch should not be changed within the first 2 days of the first application or of any change in dose. Adequate analgesia should be achieved using breakthrough medication as needed. Subsequent dose changes should be made according to the patient's requirement for breakthrough analgesics or follow the 'increase by 30–50%' rule; the patch strength as near to this increase as possible should be selected.

13.3 **Transdermal fentanyl**

Fentanyl is a strong mu opioid receptor agonist thought to provide analgesia through its effect on pain pathways in the thalamus. It causes less constipation than morphine and other less lipophilic opioids and may, in some patients, reduce other adverse effects such as delirium caused by other opioids (see Chapter 7).

13.3.1 **Patch technologies**

There are two preparations of transdermal fentanyl patch. The original Durogesic® fentanyl reservoir patch is now off patent and has been replaced by a generic reservoir patch. Two new preparations, Durogesic D Trans® and Matrifen® using a matrix, are now available. Each product has patch doses of 25, 50, 75 and 100 µg/h. A patch strength of 12.5 µg/h is also available as Durogesic D Trans® (labelled as 12 µg/h), but this is only licensed for titration between larger doses, not as a starting dose. Matrifen® is also available as a 12 µg/h patch.

There are some differences between the two technologies. Trials in normal volunteers suggest equipotency of analgesic effect, however, in clinical use there is some suggestion that the reservoir and matrix patches are not interchangeable, perhaps because of difference in adhesiveness, especially in patients with sweating. It is suggested by the

Royal Pharmaceutical Society of Great Britain that products be consistently prescribed perhaps by trade name to avoid any risks for patients of under or overdosing. Generic patches are not currently labelled by dose or name. Patch sizes also differ between the products, the reservoir patches being larger, which at higher doses may make a considerable difference to whether using multiple patches is practical.

13.3.2 Indications

The licensed indications for use are in the management of chronic intractable pain due to cancer and non-malignant causes.

Clincial indications for transdermal fentanyl are intolerable side effects from other opioids, renal impairment, dysphagia, tablet phobia or poor compliance and patient choice. Contraindications are patients with unstable pain who need rapid pain control and pain unresponsive to opioids.

13.3.3 Evidence of efficacy in cancer pain

Studies have suggested that transdermal fentanyl provides at least comparable pain relief to other opioids. A pooled analysis suggests that it may provide increased pain relief compared to modified release morphine as well as reduced constipation and somnolence. Trials using a fentanyl patch as the first line strong opioid at step III of the World Health Organization (WHO) ladder have indicated that it is effective and safe but all such trials have been carried out in very closely supervised environments, for example, some of the early trials were carried out with inpatients.

Long-term follow-up of patients indicates that treatment with transdermal fentanyl is safe and acceptable and patients rarely require more than 300 µg/h with the median end dose suggested as around 100 µg/h. Some patients (12%) appear to develop site problems such as skin soreness or detachment, but this may be less with the newer matrix patch. There is some suggestion that patients using transdermal fentanyl are more satisfied with their analgesic regimen overall than those using oral morphine.

13.3.4 Commencing transdermal fentanyl

For most patients, transdermal fentanyl is used as a second or third line strong opioid. Discussion about the optimum conversion ratio for calculating the starting dose of fentanyl is ongoing. In Germany, a ratio of morphine to fentanyl of 100:1 is widely used whilst manufacturer guidelines used in the USA and other countries use a more conservative ratio of 150:1. Skaer (2006) suggests that there is evidence in the literature on the management of cancer pain for the less conservative conversion and suggests an algorithm using the equivalance between 60 mg/day oral morphine and a 25 µg/h fentanyl patch, with titration upwards at 24 h if required. Twycross and colleagues (2003) suggest equating the equivalent 24 h diamorphine mg/day dose to the µg/h fentanyl patch dose (i.e. 100 mg/24 h diamorphine = 100 µg/h fentanyl patch).

In 10% of patients, a physical (flu-like symptoms, diarrhoea, nausea, rhinorrhoea) and/or depressive opioid withdrawal syndrome occurs on changing from morphine to transdermal fentanyl. This is short lived (usually a few days) and easily treated by the use of normal release morphine when symptoms occur. Most patients will need to reduce their laxatives and some patients develop diarrhoea, which can be controlled by small, reducing doses of morphine.

13.3.5 **Increasing the dose**

Dose increases should be made by calculating the patient's requirement for breakthrough anlagesics but more commonly, because patients tend to underuse their breakthrough analgesics, are in patch dose steps, that is, 25 then 50 then 75 and 100 µg/h. At lower doses this means a 100% increase in dose, which may not be appropriate. The 12 µg/h patch may have a role in providing smaller increments. At higher doses, consideration should be given to increments of 30–50%, for example, 200 then 275 µg/h. Smaller dose increments may provide little additional analgesic benefit although there is no research evidence to support this.

13.3.6 **Stopping transdermal fentanyl**

Transdermal fentanyl may need to be discontinued because a patient has rapidly changing pain or because of side effects. The elimination half-life is 12–22 h once a patch is removed. Whilst there are no specific guidelines, appropriate strategies should be employed depending on whether or not a patient's pain is under control. For a patient whose pain is controlled, patches should be removed 12 h before commencing an alternative opioid, and an adequate dose of normal release oral opioid prescribed for breakthrough pain.

In a patient whose pain is not controlled, a 30% increase in the dose of alternative opioid should be incorporated and a 4-hourly dose of normal release opioid given as the patch is removed and as required. The daily regimen of the alternative opioid should be commenced about 12 h after removing the transdermal patch. It is vital to review the patient regularly during this changeover period.

13.3.7 **Managing breakthrough pain**

Patients need access to a normal release opioid for exacerbations of pain. This could be any opioid preparation titrated to effect (see Chapter 14). There are two oral transmucosal fentanyl preparations; one a lozenge and one a sublingual tablet currently in trial.

13.3.8 **The terminal phase**

A patient may continue using transdermal patches until they die. It is common practice to manage any increase in pain with the addition of

Table 13.1 The transdermal buprenorphine range

	Hourly dose (μg/h)	Daily dose (mg)	Total dose (mg)	Patch area (cm^2)	Approximate equivalence (oral)
Transtec® 35	35	0.8	20	25	30–60 mg morphine/day
Transtec® 52.5	52.5	1.2	30	37.5	90 mg morphine/day
Transtec® 70	70	1.6	40	50	120 mg morphine/day
BuTrans® 5	5	0.12	5	6.25	30–60 mg codeine/day
BuTrans® 10	10	0.24	10	12.5	60–120 mg codeine/day
BuTrans® 20	20	0.48	20	25	120–240 mg codeine/day

subcutaneous opioids via a syringe driver. Alternatively, the patch may be removed and the patient's opioid requirement replaced by subcutaneous opioids via a syringe driver.

13.4 Transdermal buprenorphine

Buprenorphine is a mixed mu receptor agonist and kappa receptor antagonist. It causes less constipation than morphine.

13.4.1 Patch technology

Buprenorphine is incorporated into an adhesive polymer matrix, which controls the release of the drug by diffusion. There are two preparations, Transtec®, lasting 4 days, and BuTrans®, lasting 7 days. (See Table 13.1).

13.4.2 Licensed indications

Transtec and BuTrans patches are licensed for moderate to severe cancer pain and severe pain not responding to non-opioid analgesics. They are not suitable for the treatment of acute pain. Both preparations are controlled drugs.

13.4.3 Evidence of efficacy in cancer pain

There have been three double-blind, randomized placebo-controlled trials of Transtec® patches in patients with chronic pain, some due to cancer. In one study of 151 patients (55% with cancer), given placebo, Transtec® 35, 52.5 or 70 μg/h applied for 9 days, Bohme and colleagues reported that there were no significant differences in pain relief or breakthrough use, but more patients using Transtec® reported good or complete pain relief, milder pain intensity and uninterrupted sleep. In another study of 154 patients (77% with cancer), given placebo,

Transtec® 35, 52.5 or 70 μg/h applied for 15 days, Sittl and colleagues (2003) noted the proportion of patients needing one or less break-through doses was significantly better for 35 (37%) and 52.5 (48%) patches but not 70 μg/h (33%) compared to placebo (16%). The mean daily dose of rescue analgesic was significantly lower among all patients using Transtec® (0.3 versus 0.7 mg/day with placebo). The third study of 137 patients (33% with cancer) by Sorge and Sittl (2004) had a 5-day run-in, then 15 days of placebo or Transtec® 35 μg/h, and showed a reduction in sublingual buprenorphine use of 41% for placebo and 61% for Transtec® in the cancer pain group, however, this was not a statis-tically significant difference.

An open-label, uncontrolled follow-up study in 239 patients (56% with cancer) with chronic pain demonstrated pain control rated as at least satisfactory by 90% of patients using Transtec® for a mean duration of 7.5 months. Likar and colleagues (2006) suggested the patch was well tolerated, the most common systemic side effects being nausea (9%), dizziness (5%), vomiting (4%) and constipation (4%). Local reactions included erythema (12%) and pruritus (11%).

There have been no studies examining BuTrans® in cancer pain. Studies showing efficacy of the 7-day patch in treating chronic osteoarthritic, low back and non-malignant pains compared to sublingual buprenorphine tablets, paracetamol/oxycodone and placebo patches have been presented as abstracts but not yet in peer reviewed journals.

13.4.4 **Starting transdermal buprenorphine**

Buprenorphine absorption with the first patch provides a minimal effective concentration after 12–24 h and a maximal concentration after 57–59 h. For Transtec® patches the manufacturer suggests starting with 35 μg/h if the patient has previously been taking a weak opioid. A potency ratio of 70:1 with oral morphine was originally recommended but data from a retrospective study suggest the ratio might be 100:1 or above.

13.4.5 **Increasing the dose**

If patients require more than two breakthrough doses per 24 h, the patch dose should be increased by 30–50%, if pain is opioid responsive. The manufacturer recommends using no more than two patches at a time for either formulation.

13.4.6 **Stopping transdermal buprenorphine**

The principles of stopping transdermal buprenorphine are the same as for stopping transdermal fentanyl; the differences are the longer elimination half-life of approximately 30 h, the partial agonist effect and the potential interference in binding of alternative opioids due to high receptor affinity. While there is no specific evidence to guide practice at present, following the principles outlined for fentanyl but delaying starting alternative opioids for 18–24 h would be reasonable. Regular review is particularly important during a changeover period.

13.4.7 **Breakthrough pain**

Theoretically, as buprenorphine is a partial agonist with high receptor affinity, using alternative opioids for breakthrough pain might be problematic. There has been one open label study of 29 patients with cancer showing that intravenous morphine reduced pain by at least 50% in 83% of 106 breakthrough events, suggesting morphine is an effective medication for breakthrough use.

Sublingual buprenorphine has a higher incidence of side effects than the transdermal formulation, and anecdotally oral morphine, oxycodone and hydromorphone have been successfully used as breakthrough medication.

13.4.8 **The terminal phase**

There is currently no evidence to guide practice in the terminal phase. It is not clear how effective adding a syringe driver with an additional subcutaneous opioid will be, given the partial agonist action of buprenorphine. Removing the buprenorphine patch and switching to an alternative opioid will also be complicated given the long elimination half-life. Careful titration will be needed in either scenario over 24–48 h.

13.4.9 **Clinical cautions**

The same site should not be used for 3–4 weeks as after a 14-day rest period in healthy volunteers, same site use resulted in almost doubled plasma levels. Similar drug delivery occurs when a patch is applied to the upper outer arm, upper chest, upper back or the side of the chest but is 26% higher when applied to the upper back compared to the side of the chest.

Respiratory depression is not seen in clinically recommended doses but should it occur, due to buprenorphine's high receptor affinity, naloxone only partially reverses its effects. Naloxone doses may need to be increased and an infusion may be required due to the long duration of action of buprenorphine.

13.5 **Alternatives to morphine**

Transdermal opioids may be useful in patients who have difficulty swallowing oral medication or where patch delivery is preferred or might aid compliance. Patients must have stable pain, so that transdermal opioid delivery is not an alternative to morphine in patients who require rapid pain control and therefore need titration with normal release opioids. In patients with stable pain, and particularly for patients where opioid induced constipation remains a problem despite adequate management, they provide an alternative.

Like all the other opioids discussed in previous chapters, current evidence suggests transdermal buprenorphine may be an alternative to low dose morphine and transdermal fentanyl an alternative to morphine, but neither are superior as analgesics.

Key references

Bohme, K. and Likar, R. (2003). Efficacy and tolerability of a new opioid analgesic formulation, buprenorphine transdermal therapeutic system (TDS), in the treatment of patients with chronic pain. A randomized, double-blind, placebo-controlled study. *Pain Clinic*, **15**, 193–202.

Budd, K. (2002). Buprenorphine: a review. In *Evidence based medicine in practice*, pp.1–24. Hayward Medical Communications, Newmarket.

Clark, A.J., Ahmedzai, S.H., Allan, L.G., Camacho, F., Horbay, G.L.A., Richarz, U., *et al.* (2004). Efficacy and safety of transdermal fentanyl and sustained-release oral morphine in patients with cancer and chronic non-cancer pain. *Cur. Med. Res. Opin.,* **20**, 1419–28.

Ellershaw, J.E., Kinder, C., Aldridge, J., Allison, M. and Smith, J.C. (2002). Care of the dying: is pain control compromised or enhanced by continuation of the fentanyl transdermal patch in the dying phase? *J. Pain Symptom Manage.*, **24**, 398–403.

Likar, R., Kayser, H. and Sittl, R. (2006). Long-term management of chronic pain with transdermal buprenorphine: a multicenter, open-label, follow-up study in patients from three short-term clinical trials. *Clin. Ther.*, **28**, 943–52.

Mercadante, S., Villari, P., Ferrera, P., Porzio, G., Aielli, F., Verna, L., *et al.* (2006). Safety and effectiveness of intravenous morphine for episodic breakthrough pain in patients receiving transdermal buprenorphine. *J. Pain Symptom Manage.*, **32**, 175–9.

Sittl, R., Griessinger, N. and Likar, R. (2003). Analgesic efficacy and tolerability of transdermal buprenorphine in patients with inadequately controlled chronic pain related to cancer and other disorders: a multicenter, randomized, double-blind, placebo-controlled trial. *Clin. Ther.,* **25**, 150–68.

Skaer, T.L. (2006). Transdermal opioids for cancer pain. *Health Qual. Life Outcomes*, **4**, 24.

Sorge, J. and Sittl, R. (2004). Transdermal buprenorphine in the treatment of chronic pain: results of a phase III, multicenter, randomized, double-blind, placebo-controlled study, *Clin. Ther.*, **26**, 1808–20.

Twycross, R., Wilcock, A., Charlesworth, S. and Dickman, A. (2003). *Palliative care formulary*. 2nd edn. Radcliffe Publishing, Oxford.

Chapter 14

Other routes of opioid administration

Giovambattista Zeppetella

> **Key points**
>
> - The oral route is the commonest route of opioid administration.
> - In some instances, clinical circumstances make a switch to an alternative route of administration desirable.
> - Common alternative routes include oral transmucosal, rectal, inhaled and topical administration.
> - The evidence base for alternatives to the oral route is often from case reports; the strongest evidence is for oral transmucosal fentanyl citrate in the management of breakthrough pain.
> - There are few non-oral licensed preparations available and most use is off-label.

14.1 Introduction

When prescribing opioids for cancer pain, the oral route is preferred often because it is convenient and usually inexpensive. Although oral opioids often can be continued up until death there are circumstances when this is not feasible or desirable. A number of factors may contribute to choosing an alternative route of administration including

- Patient related, for example, dysphagia, nausea, vomiting, malabsorption, weakness, patient preference.
- Pain related, for example, speed of onset, duration and predictability.
- Opioid related, for example, pharmacokinetic and pharmacodynamic profile.

Non-oral opioids may be used for titration, maintenance and breakthrough pain. When changing the route of administration and not the drug, the dose of the drug is usually adjusted; this is particularly important when switching between oral and parenteral routes if the opioid undergoes extensive first pass metabolism. Patients will often accept an alternative to the oral route, but for this to be successful the alternative route should be simple, safe, effective and free of adverse effects. This chapter will consider the benefits and disadvantages of the transmucosal and topical opioid administration routes.

14.2 **Oral transmucosal route**

The oral mucosa is easily accessible and a convenient site for drug delivery. Oral transmucosal delivery is non-invasive and less threatening to patients than other routes of administration such as intravenous or intramuscular administration; furthermore, it does not require technical equipment, expertise, preparation and supervision. Some opioids have a bitter taste and it may be difficult to know how much drug is swallowed and how much is absorbed transmucosally. In addition, this route may not be appropriate in patients with cognitive impairment.

The oral transmucosal surfaces can be used to deliver a number of different types of dosage form, such as bioadhesive systems (tablets or patches), fast melting tablets, liquid drug-filled capsules or sprays. The drugs best suited to oral transmucosal administration are those that are potent, lipophilic, and are ionized at physiological pH; the longer they are in contact with the mucosa the better their chance of absorption. The buccal and sublingual tissues are the primary focus for drug delivery via the oral mucosa because they are more permeable than the tissues in other areas of the mouth.

14.2.1 **Sublingual**

The thickness of the epithelium of the sublingual mucosa is 100–200 μm, which makes it more permeable than the remainder of the oral mucosa. The area is highly vascularised and therefore drugs that can be administered in this way have direct access to the systemic circulation.

The only drug currently licensed for administration by this route is buprenorphine, a highly lipophilic and long-acting opioid. Sublingual buprenorphine's onset of action is approximately 30 min and the duration of action is 6–9 h which might make it suitable for maintenance opioid therapy but not for breakthrough pain. Although this has been reported, buprenorphine is currently most commonly used as a transdermal matrix patch formulation (see Chapter 13).

There are reports in the literature of other opioids such as morphine, fentanyl, alfentanil, sufentanil and diamorphine being administered sublingually, often in the management of breakthrough pain, but results have been variable. In most cases, the commercially available injection is used. Only small doses can be easily accommodated and holding the dose in the mouth is inconvenient; if any is swallowed that portion must be treated as an oral dose and subject to first pass metabolism.

14.2.2 Buccal

The buccal mucosa, like the sublingual mucosa, offers a convenient, accessible and generally well-accepted route of administration. The buccal mucosa is thicker (500–600 µm) and less permeable than the sublingual area so that bioavailability is less, however, the expanse of smooth muscle and relatively immobile mucosa make it more desirable for retentive systems.

The only preparation currently licensed for administration by this route is oral transmucosal fentanyl citrate (OTFC), a fentanyl-impregnated lozenge developed specifically for the management of breakthrough pain, which is dissolved by gentle rubbing against the buccal mucosa. A number of trials have confirmed the efficacy, safety and tolerability of OTFC, including two randomized controlled studies and a long-term follow-up study. The results of clinical trials suggest the successful dose of OTFC cannot be predicted from the regularly scheduled daily opioid dose; it is therefore recommended that each patient is titrated to the dose that produces adequate analgesia and minimal adverse effects.

14.2.3 New transmucosal developments

A new development soon to be introduced into clinical practice is a fentanyl oravescent tablet that disperses quickly in the mouth without chewing or the need for water. This preparation, which can be used either buccally or sublingually, contains an additional pH-adjusting substance, in combination with the effervescent technology, for promoting buccal absorption of drugs. This results in a rapid initial rise in serum levels and, compared to OTFC, a faster more complete absorption. Other developments include an alfentanil buccal patch and several sublingual fentanyl spray preparations. All of these preparations are being developed for the management of breakthrough pain.

14.3 Rectal transmucosal opioids

Rectal administration is, in general, a safe, inexpensive and effective route for delivery of opioids. Because the rectal wall is thin and its blood supply rich, the drug can be readily absorbed, however, the pharmacology of rectally administered medications relates not only to the medication but also to the suppository base, additives, drug ionization, absorptive surface of the rectum, and rectal health.

Several opioids may be formulated as rectal preparations, including morphine, oxycodone, hydromorphone and methadone. Commercial availability may vary across countries and in some settings the normal release tablet is placed into a gelatine capsule to make a suppository; a modified release morphine hydrogel suppository is available in some countries. The dose administered and the duration of analgesia is usually the same as for the oral dose. Although rectal opioids can be administered simply by unskilled carers, there may be reluctance in some cultures to using this route. Furthermore, prolonged use should be avoided, as it may be uncomfortable. Rectal administration can provide quick pain relief, however, absorption, and therefore pain relief, may be variable.

14.4 **Inhaled transmucosal opioids**

The respiratory tract extends from the nasal orifices to the periphery of the lungs. Drug administration by this route is complicated by the complexity of the anatomical structure of the human respiratory system and the influence on drug deposition exerted by respiration. Despite this, the inhalation route is of increasing interest for both local and systemic drug delivery, including macromolecular biopharmaceuticals, such as peptides, proteins and gene therapies; less is known about analgesia associated with nebulized or aerosol delivery. Both pulmonary and nasal routes have been used for opioid administration, however, these routes may not be useful for patients with respiratory disease, or those who are extremely ill, comatose or cognitively impaired.

14.4.1 **Nebulized opioids**

The lung provides a large surface area, thin absorptive mucosal membrane and good blood supply; all of which favour systemic absorption. Although inhaled medications are commonly used in general medicine, there are few reports of opioids for pain, other than in the management of postoperative pain where morphine, fentanyl, diamorphine, hydromorphone and codeine have all been investigated. There are few data on nebulized opioids for pain control in patients with cancer; one case report has described the analgesic effects of nebulized fentanyl.

Although nebulizers are non-invasive and generally acceptable to patients, they can be cumbersome, noisy and an inefficient way of delivering medication. Also a bitter taste has been reported with morphine, whilst cough and nasal pruritus have been reported with fentanyl. Bioavailability via this route is a subject of debate and there is evidence to suggest that nebulized morphine is poorly absorbed. It may be that other more potent or lipophilic opioids could be administered appropriately by this route for systemic delivery, but thus far, variations in absorption of inhaled opioids remain a limiting factor for the use of inhaled opioids for pain control. Newer delivery systems that provide more efficient absorption are in development for the management of breakthrough pain; both morphine and fentanyl have been used.

14.4.2 **Nasal opioids**

The nasal cavity is a potential target for the administration of systemically acting opioids as, like other transmucosal routes, the nasal cavity is readily accessible, has a highly permeable mucosa, a high total blood flow and avoids first pass metabolism. There are two primary limitations of intranasal drug delivery, namely, mucosal irritation and poor bioavailability. To improve bioavailability, bioadhesive drug delivery systems have been used. These drug delivery systems have the ability to control the rate of drug clearance from the nasal cavity and protect the drug from enzymatic degradation in nasal secretions, thus improving drug absorption.

The literature contains a number of reports describing the nasal administration of opioids, either as a dry powder or dissolved in water or saline. The pharmacokinetics of intranasal fentanyl, alfentanil, oxycodone, buprenorphine and butorphanol administered to healthy volunteers have been published. There are also reports exploring the role of intranasal opioids in the postoperative setting. Morphine, hydromorphone, methadone, fentanyl and alfentanil have all been delivered nasally in palliative care settings, often in the management of breakthrough pain. The nasal route can allow self-administration of opioid with rapid onset of action ideally suited to the characteristics of most breakthrough pains. A major disadvantage with the currently available opioid preparations is the relatively small volume of drug the nose is able to accommodate. Larger volumes pass into the back of the throat and are swallowed, and thus subject to first pass metabolism. More concentrated preparations are currently being tested by this route in clinical trials.

14.5 **Topical opioids**

There may be instances when successful analgesia is best achieved by direct administration of the opioid onto or near the painful area. The potential advantages of a local delivery system include optimizing opioid concentration at the site of pain, lower plasma opioid levels with potentially fewer adverse effects, and fewer drug interactions.

All classes of opioid receptors have now been demonstrated on peripheral nerve terminals, and are similar to the population of receptors found in the central nervous system. Opioid receptors are not evident in normal tissue but become detectable within minutes to hours after the start of inflammation, following increased production within the dorsal root ganglion and axonal transportation towards the nerve terminals. Two of the commonest applications of local delivery are intra-articular opioids and opioids applied to malignant and non-malignant ulcers.

14.5.1 **Intra-articular administration**

The demonstration of peripheral opioid receptors as well as opioid peptides in inflamed synovium supports the concept of peripheral opioid analgesia and several studies have explored the analgesic effects of postoperative intra-articular morphine. A systematic review by Kalso and colleagues (2002) indicates that low doses of morphine administered by this route are effective and can last up to 24 h and that this effect could be dose dependent. Effective doses are relatively low and produce plasma levels incapable of producing a systemic effect, hence adverse effects are uncommon. Studies which show no effect have often demonstrated a lack of tissue inflammation. There have been reports of other opioids including fentanyl, sufentanil, buprenorphine and pethidine, used successfully by this route.

14.5.2 **Malignant and non-malignant ulcers**

Painful skin ulcers are a common problem in the palliative care setting and systemic analgesics are often of limited benefit. Current evidence in the form of case reports and small controlled trials supports the use of topical opioids. Morphine is the most commonly used opioid reported, although diamorphine, fentanyl, oxycodone and pethidine have also been used. Usually the chosen opioid has been mixed in a carrier such as intrasite gel, although where the wound was infected sulphadiazine cream and metronidazole gel have been used. Most studies have applied opioids to open wounds although analgesia after application to an area of inflamed intact skin has also been reported.

The effective dose of topical opioids appears to be relatively low and patients describe analgesia, the duration of which appears longer than is seen with the corresponding opioid delivered systemically. Despite patients taking a wide range of systemic opioid doses, some reports describe analgesia lasting for up to 2 days. Further work is required to confirm these preliminary findings.

14.5.3 **Other topical administration**

Opioids have reportedly been delivered topically, intraperitoneally, dentally, perineurally and intrapleurally in other situations including mucositis, dental pain, vesical pain and wound pain.

14.6 **Other routes**

The vagina has also been used for transmucosal administration for the management of pain; both morphine and fentanyl have been administered, in some cases for prolonged periods of time.

Table 14.1 Summary of advantages and disadvantages of oral, transmucosal and topical drug administration

Route	Advantages	Disadvantages	Not recommended
Oral	Easy to administer Well tolerated Inexpensive Modified release preparations available	Lowest bioavailability Slow absorption for some breakthrough pains	Nausea, vomiting, bowel obstruction, dysphagia, coma
Buccal	Easily accessible Convenient High bioavailability Fast absorption	Limited drug formulations available No modified release formulations Bitter taste	Oral pathology
Rectal	Easy to administer Generally safe Inexpensive Modified release preparations available	Variable absorption Not always tolerated or acceptable	Diarrhoea, haemorrhoids, anal fissure
Pulmonary	Easy to administer Convenient Large area for absorption	No specific formulations available Variable bioavailability	Respiratory disease, coma or cognitive impairment
Nasal	Easily accessible Easy to administer	Small surface area Mucosal irritation Variable bioavailability No specific formulations available	Nasal pathology
Topical	Direct application to site of pain Few systemic effects	No specific formulations available Still under development	Necrotic or sloughy wound

14.7 **Summary**

Successful pharmacotherapy of pain often depends on the mode of drug delivery. Alternatives to the oral route can offer advantages in the management of cancer pain, particularly when the oral route is not available or the characteristic of the pain suggests that it may not be suitable. There is very limited information published on the clinical use of the rectal, sublingual, buccal and inhalational routes in patients with cancer pain. Available pharmacokinetic data and limited clinical experience suggest the specific application of these routes in some clinical situations; in most cases, medication for breakthrough pain is delivered by these routes although maintenance opioid therapy for short periods has also been reported.

All of the routes mentioned may be useful in patients in whom the oral route must be bypassed because of bowel obstruction, severe emesis or severe dysphagia. The buccal, sublingual and inhalational routes will not be useful in patients with severe cognitive impairment or comatose states, whereas the rectal route will not be useful in patients with diarrhoea, colostomy, haemorrhoids or anal fissures. In relatively few cases have products been developed specifically to be administered by the non-oral route; in most cases, the intravenous preparation is administered and without the appropriate studies these routes of administration are likely to remain 'off-label' (Table 14.1).

Key references

Dale, O. (2006). Opioids via other routes. In: *Cancer-related breakthrough pain.* Oxford Pain Management Library (ed. A. Davies), pp. 73–82. Oxford University Press, Oxford.

Kalso, E., Smith, L., McQuay, H.J. and Moore, R.A. (2002). No pain no gain: clinical excellence and scientific vigor—lessons from IA morphine. *Pain,* **98**, 269–75.

Walker, G., Wilcock, A., Manderson, C., Weller, R. and Crosby, V. (2003). The acceptability of different routes of administration of analgesia for breakthrough pain. *Palliat. Med.,* **17**, 219–21.

Warren, D.E. (1996). Practical use of rectal medications in palliative care. *J. Pain Symptom Manage.,* **11**, 378–87.

Webster, L.R. (2006). Fentanyl buccal tablets. *Exp. Opin. Investig. Drugs,* **15**, 1469–73.

Zeppetella, G. (2004). Topical opioids for painful skin ulcers. Do they work? *Eur. J. Palliat. Care,* **11**, 93–6.

Zeppetella, G. and Ribeiro, M.D.C. (2006). Opioids for the management of breakthrough (episodic) pain in cancer patients. *Cochrane Database Syst. Rev.*, **1**, CD004311.

Zeppetella, G. (2006) Oral transmucosal opioid drugs. In: *Cancer-related breakthrough pain*. Oxford Pain Management Library (ed. A. Davies), pp. 57–71. Oxford University Press, Oxford.

Chapter 15

Spinal opioids

Karen H. Simpson and Ganesan Baranidharan

Key points

- Spinal opioids mediate their main actions via mu receptors in the brain and in the substantia gelatinosa within the dorsal horn of the spinal cord.
- Neuraxial opioids can be very useful when the World Health Organization (WHO) analgesic ladder fails to provide adequate analgesia or leads to unmanageable adverse effects.
- Intrathecal drug delivery has advantages over epidural drug delivery such as low dose requirements and fewer longer-term complications.
- Careful patient selection is crucial and should include intrathecal test dosing.
- Multidisciplinary team work and good post-procedure support are essential for the ongoing management of intrathecal drug delivery to optimize analgesia and manage adverse events.

15.1 Introduction

Opioids have been used by a variety of routes to manage pain since the ninth century. After the discovery of spinal opioid receptors in 1976, Behar and Wong first used spinal opioids in humans in 1979. Almost 90% of cancer pain can be treated by the WHO analgesic ladder; most other patients can be managed by parenteral administration of opioids and co-analgesics. Only about 2% of patients with cancer pain need more invasive management using neuraxial opioids.

15.1.1 Indications for spinal opioids

- Escalating opioid requirements.
- Pain not amenable to opioid switching.
- Unacceptable/intolerable side effects from systemic opioids.
- Good response to intrathecal test dose.

15.1.2 **Contraindications to spinal opioids**

- Patient refusal.
- Head and neck pain (intracerebroventricular drug administration may be helpful).
- High cranial or spinal cerebrospinal fluid (CSF) pressure or poor CSF flow.
- Impending spinal cord compression.
- Local or systemic infection.
- Uncorrectable bleeding disorders or the need to continue anticoagulant therapies.
- Allergy to currently available intrathecal drugs.
- Inadequate post-treatment support available in primary or secondary care.

15.2 **Routes of spinal drug administration**

Drugs can be delivered via either epidural or intrathecal catheters; both have advantages and disadvantages (Table 15.1). The main issue that separates the techniques is the practical difficulty due to catheter fibrosis and higher dose requirement that often occurs with epidural drug delivery. Therefore, the intrathecal route may be preferred to the epidural for longer-term use.

15.3 **Spinal opioid mechanisms**

Spinal opioids act via the mu receptors located in the substantia gelatinosa of the spinal cord dorsal horn; they also spread intracranially via CSF flow to act in the brain. Morphine produces a dose dependant presynaptic inhibition of neurotransmitter release from small primary afferent fibres. It causes hyperpolarization of postsynaptic neurones that suppress nociceptive stimuli.

15.4 **Choice of opioids**

Currently there is a wide choice of opioids available for spinal use. The ability to deliver these drugs effectively intrathecally depends on:

- Age.
- General medical condition.
- Body habitus.
- Intra-abdominal pressure.
- Disease burden.

Table 15.1 Relative risks and benefits for intrathecal (ITDD) and epidural drug delivery

	ITDD	Epidural drug delivery
Infection rate	Same as epidural	Same as intrathecal
Pain relief	Better for long term	Good for very short term
Dose/volume infused	Low	High
Pump refills	Less frequent	More frequent
Side effects	Few	More
Technical complications First 20 days Long term	25% (CSF leak) 5%	8% 55%
Catheter occlusion and fibrosis	Low	High (50%)
Effect of epidural metastasis	Less	More
Suitable for management at home	More suitable (Low volume infusions)	Less suitable

- Characteristics of CSF volume, constitution and flow.
- Spinal catheter tip position.
- Physical, chemical and pharmacological properties of the opioid.
- Opioid dose needed.
- Available formulations and their specific gravity and baricity.
- Co-administration of other spinal analgesics, for example, clonidine, local anaesthetics or baclofen.

15.4.1 **Morphine**

Morphine is a hydrophilic opioid with low lipid solubility. Lipid solubility is expressed relative to morphine; with morphine having a solubility of 1. It has a slow onset (30–60 min) with a long duration of action (12–24 h), after spinal delivery. Spinal morphine is 5–10 times more potent than with the intravenous route. Owing to its high water solubility and rostral spread in CSF, it can give pain relief at a higher dermatomal level than the catheter tip. Its use has reduced due to the potential for formation of catheter-related granulomas probably associated with slow, concentrated morphine infusions. The catheter tip should be positioned with radiological screening in the lumbar thecal sac posterior to the cord, to reduce drug pooling. A dilute morphine concentration should be used with vigilant follow-up for any symptoms or signs of neurological compromise that could indicate a granuloma. Magnetic resonance imaging (MRI) scanning may be needed (see below).

15.4.2 Hydromorphone

Hydromorphone has a lipid solubility of 1.4 with an onset of 20–30 min and an intermediate duration of action (6–12 h). It is five times more potent spinally than with the intravenous route. Thus far, animal studies have not been associated with catheter tip inflammatory masses.

15.4.3 Fentanyl and sufentanil

Fentanyl and sufentanil are both highly lipid soluble, with a short duration of action (2–4 h) and a rapid onset (10–20 min) when used spinally. Owing to their low CSF solubility, these drugs are equipotent when given spinally or intravenously.

15.4.4 Buprenorphine

Buprenorphine is a partial opioid agonist and antagonist; it is not an ideal agent for spinal analgesia.

15.4.5 Pethidine

Pethidine is lipophilic (fat soluble); it has a 4–8 h duration of action. Spinally it is 1–2 times more potent than after intravenous dosing. It also has some local anaesthetic characteristics. It is eliminated more rapidly from the CSF than morphine and offers no clear advantages.

15.4.6 Methadone

Methadone is lipophilic. It has a low CSF solubility. It has high dose requirement, increased side effects and inferior quality of analgesia and is therefore usually not used as a spinal opioid.

15.5 Adjuvant drugs

As disease progresses, pain management can become challenging. Combining a spinal opioid with a drug from a different class increases the chance of effective pain control and may reduce side effects. Drugs have been used spinally to

- Reduce neuronal excitability
  - Local anaesthetics, for example, bupivacaine, lidocaine
  - Ketamine
  - Anti-inflammatory drugs, for example, ketorolac, diclofenac.
- Increase neuronal inhibition
  - Clonidine
  - Neostigmine.

15.5.1 Ziconotide

This is a new non-opioid, non-local anaesthetic spinal agent that has been developed for the treatment of severe chronic pain. It is a synthetic cone snail peptide analogue (w-conotoxin M-VII-A). It is a neuronal specific calcium channel blocker that acts by blocking N-type voltage sensitive calcium channels and is not associated with granuloma formation. Clinical experience with ziconotide is still early and limited, but it may have a role in neuropathic pain management. It requires careful and slow dose titration.

15.6 Choice of spinal drugs

Taking all factors into consideration, an algorithm has been developed by the Polyanalgesic Consensus Group to suggest logical choices of spinal drugs; this will change as new data emerges and the recommendations will probably be updated in 2007 (Figure 15.1).

15.7 Techniques for ITDD

The choice of external or internal intrathecal drug delivery system (ITDD) system depends on the patient's life expectancy, available health care professionals' skills, resources and local infrastructures. Patients usually require sedation or general anaesthesia for spinal catheter and/or pump implants. A single dose of antibiotic is given immediately prior to surgery, but antibiotics should not be used routinely after implants. An intrathecal catheter is placed under

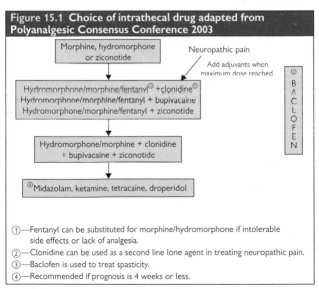

Figure 15.1 Choice of intrathecal drug adapted from Polyanalgesic Consensus Conference 2003

Morphine, hydromorphone or ziconotide

Neuropathic pain

Add adjuvants when maximum dose reached

Hydromorphone/morphine/fentanyl[1] +clonidine[2]
Hydromorphone/morphine/fentanyl + bupivacaine
Hydromorphone/morphine/fentanyl + ziconotide

Hydromorphone/morphine + clonidine + bupivacaine + ziconotide

[4]Midazolam, ketamine, tetracaine, droperidol

BACLOFEN

[1]—Fentanyl can be substituted for morphine/hydromorphone if intolerable side effects or lack of analgesia.
[2]—Clonidine can be used as a second line lone agent in treating neuropathic pain.
[3]—Baclofen is used to treat spasticity.
[4]—Recommended if prognosis is 4 weeks or less.

Figure 15.1 is reproduced with permission from Hassenbusch, S.J. (2004). Polyanalgesic consensus conference 2003: an update on the management of pain by intraspinal drug delivery-report of an expert panel. *Journal of Pain Symptom Management*. **27**, 540–63.

strict aseptic conditions using radiological screening in an operating room. The catheter is anchored to the supraspinous ligament to prevent migration or dislodging. The catheter is then tunnelled to the abdomen for connection to an external pump or to a subcutaneously placed fully implantable pump in the abdominal wall.

15.7.1 **ITDD systems**

A fully implanted system should usually be used only if the patient is expected to survive for at least 3 months; otherwise an external system is needed. The choice of appropriate ITDD system can be supported by using a simple algorithm (Figure 15.2); however, each case still needs to be individually judged in terms of benefits and risks.

External pumps must be able to deliver small infusion volumes accurately. Pumps should be small, lightweight, easy to handle and tamper proof having long-term memory storage and a battery alarm. Most pumps used in the management of acute pain can be used; those with a large volume cassette are better, as changes to drug infusions must be kept to a minimum to reduce the risk of infection. There are also disposable pumps that deliver at a set rate; some have a bolus facility.

Internal pumps are placed in a subcutaneous pocket either in the abdomen or buttock. The injection port can be accessed percutaneously for refills. Some internal pumps use a compressed gas to give a constant rate infusion. Their infusion rate may be altered by changes in barometric pressure, for example, during scuba diving and air travel, and patients need to be made aware of this. Other fully programmable pumps allow full control of the rate of infusion; these are programmed using an external telemetric controller. Medtronic Synchromed pumps can also give a patient controlled bolus dose if needed. Fully programmable pumps are more expensive and more training is needed for their management. Electromagnetic interference (EMI) is an energy field generated by equipment found at home, work, medical or public environments. Most EMI normally encountered will not affect the operation of fully implanted pumps. Patients can safely go through airport scanners and travel by air. MRI will temporarily stop the pump motor's rotor due to the magnetic field of the MRI scanner and suspend the drug infusion, thus triggering the pump alarm. Prior to MRI, the pump should be emptied and turned off and a plan for continuing therapy should be in place. Pump function should be tested pre- and post-MRI. An internal pump should be removed after death as the pumps can explode if cremation is planned, or if local environmental regulations mandate removal.

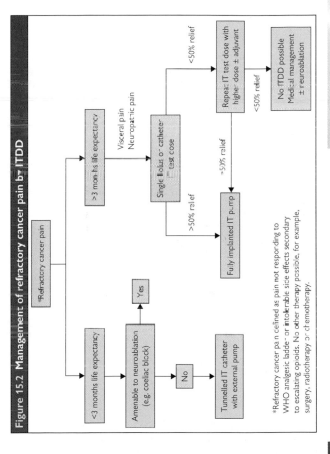

Figure 15.2 Management of refractory cancer pain by ITDD

*Refractory cancer pain

<3 months life expectancy

Amenable to neuroablation (e.g. coeliac block)

Yes

No

Tunnelled IT catheter with external pump

>3 months life expectancy

Visceral pain
Neuropathic pain

Single bolus or catheter test dose

>50% relief

<50% relief

Fully implanted IT pump

>50% relief

Repeat IT test dose with higher dose ± adjuvant

<50% relief

No ITDD possible
Medical management
± neuroablation

*Refractory cancer pain defined as pain not responding to
WHO analgesic ladder or intolerable side effects secondary
to escalating opioids. No other therapy possible, for example,
surgery, radiotherapy or chemotherapy.

Table 15.2 Spinal opioid dose conversion				
Drug	Oral	Parenteral	Epidural	Intrathecal
Morphine (mg)	30	10	1	0.1
Hydromorphone (mg)	5	2	0.2	0.02
Fentanyl (µg)	NA	100	50–100	5–20
Sufentanil (µg)	NA	10	10	5–10

15.7.2 **Drug conversion regimens**

Effective and safe conversion from oral/systemic opioid administration to spinal opioid analgesia can be challenging. The key aims are a smooth transition over a sensible period, with minimal withdrawal or overdose problems. This can be achieved by converting the oral opioid dose to its parenteral equivalent dose and then using one-tenth of this dose for epidural and one-hundredth for intrathecal administration (Table 15.2). Lipophilic agents such as sufentanil and fentanyl have a higher affinity for lipid tissue in the spinal cord, hence requiring a higher dose than the hydrophilic agents. Very little reaches the grey matter as most of the drug gets redistributed into the blood stream from the white matter.

15.7.3 **Continuous or bolus dosing**

Spinal opioids can be infused continuously or given as a bolus. A continuous infusion delivers drugs at a constant rate. This may lead to stable receptor occupancy and the development of tolerance; bolus use may prevent this. With continuous infusions, although analgesia may be better, more dose escalation is needed. Bolus doses may increase side effects, for example, sedation with opioids, hypotension with clonidine and motor block with local anaesthetics.

15.8 **Complications and adverse effects**

15.8.1 **Opioid related**

- Sedation.
- Nausea/vomiting.
- Urinary retention.
- Generalized pruritus.
- Respiratory depression.
- Hyperalgesia after high doses.
- Myoclonus or spinal jerking syndrome.
- Tolerance/dose escalation (this may be related to disease progression).
- Neuroendocrine suppression.

15.8.2 **Non-drug-related problems**

- Infection (local, for example, catheter track or pump pocket, epidural abscess, meningitis or systemic sepsis).
- Cerebrospinal fluid leak (headache).
- Haematoma (local or intraspinal).
- Fibrosis or granuloma at the catheter tip (may lead to cord compression).
- Catheter migration, fracture, leak, occlusion.
- Mechanical problems with the pump, for example, rotor arm stalling.
- Drug prescription/refill errors (may lead to drug withdrawal or overdose).
- Pump programming errors (may lead to drug withdrawal or overdose).

15.8.3 **Treatment failures**

Spinal opioids may be ineffective in certain situations, for example,

- Acute somatic pain/incident pain (e.g. pathological fracture).
- Continuous or intermittent visceral pain (e.g. ileus).
- Head and neck pain.
- Pain from skin ulcers.
- Some neuropathic pains.
- At the end of life.

At the end of life, pain and other symptoms can become overwhelming and ITDD is sometimes not adequate. It must be recognized if this happens and alternative therapies need to be planned in advance. In some circumstances, patients need a subcutaneous infusion as well as their ITDD device.

15.9 **Team work for successful ITDD**

Management of ITDD requires teamwork that often involves oncologists, palliative care physicians, anaesthetists, pain management specialists, specialist nurses, primary care teams, pharmacists, as well as the patient and their carers. Patients are normally identified as potentially requiring ITDD by a palliative care physician or oncologist. Early referral to the clinician providing ITDD is important. Patients can then be assessed and prepared for an internal or external pump procedure in a planned and timely manner according to Figure 15.2. A successful test dose of intrathecal opioid and/or adjuvants is needed to determine patients' suitability for ITDD. After implantation, patients are normally nursed in hospital during the initial postoperative period to manage any post-dural puncture headache, begin intrathecal dose titration and allow staged systemic dose adjustments. Following this they can be managed at home or in a palliative care unit depending upon local circumstances. Regular follow-up for dose adjustment and pump refill must be arranged with the team responsible for ITDD. The team responsible for pump placement must arrange continuous availability to deal with serious complications such as spinal bleeding or infections; robust on-call arrangements are vital.

During the terminal stages of cancer, transport becomes difficult and sometimes pump refill and dose adjustment might have to be done in the community; this requires local arrangements for training and development of expertise. It is important not to underestimate the commitment and resources needed from patients, carers and health care teams to make ITDD work well.

Key issues include

- Early referral to a pain management team if ITDD is being considered.
- Meticulous patient selection.
- Staged and clear information exchange between the medical teams, patient and carers so that properly informed consent can be given.
- Adequate investigations and preparation for catheter and/or pump implant.
- ITDD should only occur in an appropriately equipped and staffed centre with experience in the technique.
- Monitoring of pain control and adverse drug effects.
- Robust arrangements for ongoing care, drug refills and dose adjustments.
- Vigilance for and management of technical complications.
- Ongoing community support.

Key references

Burton, A.W. (2004). Epidural and intrathecal analgesia is effective in treating refractory cancer pain. *Pain Med.*, **5**, 239–47.

Hassenbusch, S.J. (2004). Polyanalgesic consensus conference 2003: an update on the management of pain by intraspinal drug delivery—report of an expert panel. *J. Pain Symptom Manage.*, **27**, 540–63.

Mercadante, S. (1999). Problems of long-term spinal opioid treatment in advanced cancer patients. *Pain*, **79**, 1–13.

Wagemans, M.F. (1997). Long-term spinal opioid therapy in terminally ill cancer pain patients. *Oncologist*, **2**, 70–5.

Chapter 16

Parenteral opioids

Jeremy R. Johnson

Key points

- Opioids can be administered parenterally when the oral route is not suitable.
- Continuous subcutaneous infusion is safe, comfortable and effective.
- Morphine and diamorphine are the commonly used World Health Organization (WHO) step III opioids.
- Other strong opioids can be given via continuous subcutaneous infusion.
- Equianalgesic tables should be used with caution.
- When converting between different formulations and routes, err on the side of caution, monitor the patient and retitrate as necessary.

16.1 Background

For most opioids, the preferred route of administration is by mouth. Oral medications are generally cheap, convenient and widely available. However, certain circumstances may preclude this route:

- Difficulty swallowing.
- Oral or pharyngeal lesions.
- Persistent nausea or vomiting.
- Poor alimentary absorption.
- Intestinal obstruction.
- Profound weakness/cachexia.
- Comatose or moribund patient.

16.2 Continuous subcutaneous infusion

Although many drugs can be given by other routes (see Chapters 14 and 15), delivery by continuous subcutaneous infusion (CSCI) is now well established in palliative care for controlling a variety of symptoms, including pain. Subcutaneous infusion is preferable to the intravenous (IV) route, is as effective as the intramuscular (IM) route and is more comfortable. Several controlled trials have reported the pharmacokinetic equivalency of CSCI to IV administration for the same preparations. CSCI is easier to manage in the community, is less expensive and can be used even when IV access is difficult. CSCI has a lower incidence of infection than for other routes of administration and the ability to infuse concentrated solutions of medications minimizes the risk of fluid overload in frail patients.

16.2.1 **Advantages of CSCI**

- Effective delivery of medication.
- Provision of 'steady state' plasma concentrations after an initial period.
- Avoids repeated (SC/IM) bolus injections (uncomfortable, and lead to 'peaks and troughs' in plasma concentration).
- System can be worn in a holster or pouch, allowing mobility and independence.
- Allows more than one drug to be given in combination.

It is preferable to keep the number of drugs combined in a CSCI to a minimum. Nevertheless, a recent survey of palliative care units has confirmed that multiple combinations are frequently employed, with good effect.

16.3 **Syringe drivers**

Syringe drivers are lightweight, portable pumps that are battery or mechanically operated and capable of delivering precise doses of medication over a fixed time period, usually 24 h. They have been widely used in palliative care for over 25 years. In the UK, the most widely used syringe drivers are the Graseby MS16A and MS26. For both of these, the rate of delivery is based on length of fluid per unit time. The MS16A (blue) delivers a rate set at mm per hour; the MS26 (green) delivers a rate set at mm per 24 h. For most 10 mL syringes used in hospital practice, 8 mL of liquid fills the barrel of the syringe to a length of 48 mm. The MS16A is then set at 2 mm per hour, the MS26 at 48 mm per 24 h. Larger volumes can be delivered via Graseby syringe drivers since they will accommodate 20 and 30 mL syringes. Other devices capable of delivering CSCIs include elastomeric balloons and cassette infusion pumps.

New legislation aimed at reducing error and tampering may require delivery rates to be measured by volume. The Graseby Advancis MS (currently a prototype) is one such device that should fulfil the requirements. To minimize potential problems or errors, it is essential that all staff setting up CSCIs should be properly trained in line with current local policies.

16.3.1 **Cautions**

Unless patients are unable to take or absorb medication via the oral route, a CSCI is unlikely to improve symptom control. It is inappropriate to commence a syringe driver solely in the hope of providing better pain control.

Patients and carers may have concerns about syringe drivers. They may find them intrusive or worry that they represent a 'last resort' signifying imminent demise. Addressing such anxieties and giving careful explanations regarding the nature and intent of the medications is vitally important.

16.3.1.1 *Commencing a continuous subcutaneous infusion— starting doses*

When starting a CSCI, the dose of opioid used will depend on the previous formulation, dose and route used. A conversion table is shown (see Table 16.1). It should be noted that such tables should be used as a guide only since there is considerable interpatient variability, depending on metabolism, tolerance, drug handling and pharmacogenetics. Furthermore, different routes may offer different 'potencies' as a result of varying bioavailability. In all cases following a change, **patients will need to be monitored and doses titrated, up or down, depending on response**. In determining a starting dose, the total amount of opioid used in the previous 24 h (background and breakthrough) needs to be taken into account before applying a conversion ratio.

When a patient is unable to take oral medication, opioids can be given subcutaneously via a syringe driver. Table 16.1 shows how to convert from oral opioids to a CSCI.

Table 16.1 Conversion from oral opioids to a CSCI		
Patient on this oral drug	Divide total 24 h oral dose by	To get this drug in syringe driver over 24 h
Oral morphine	2	Subcutaneous morphine
Oral morphine	3	Subcutaneous diamorphine
Oral morphine	3^1–4^2	Subcutaneous oxycodone
Oral morphine	15	Subcutaneous hydromorphone
Oral hydromorphone	2	Subcutaneous hydromorphone
Oral oxycodone	2	Subcutaneous oxycodone
Oral morphine	150	Subcutaneous fentanyl
Oral morphine	30	Subcutaneous alfentanil
DoH guidelines (2005)[1] and manufacturer guidelines[2] vary.		

For example, 60 mg of oral morphine in 24 h (e.g. 30 mg modified release morphine bd) will convert to a CSCI via syringe driver per 24 h with

- 30 mg of morphine,
- 20 mg of diamorphine,
- 4 mg of hydromorphone or
- 2 mg of alfentanil.

16.3.1.2 *Dose increments*

Once a CSCI has been established for at least a day and if pain is not controlled, then for most opioids the dose can be increased by 30–50%. Alternatively, the extra amount of rescue medication for breakthrough pain should be added to the previous 24 h opioid dose for the following day.

16.3.1.3 *Breakthrough pain*

For most opioids rescue medication at a dose equivalent to the 4-hourly dose, that is, one-sixth of the 24 h dose in the CSCI, should be available to the patient for oral or parenteral use. This should be given on request and repeated as necessary. Analgesics given specifically for procedural or incident/episodic pain should, however, not be added routinely to the maintenance dose of analgesia as this may lead to opioid toxicity, particularly if the patient is otherwise comfortable at rest.

16.3.1.4 *Use of the 'boost' button*

The MS26 driver is equipped with a 'boost' button. This should not be used for breakthrough pain since an adequate (i.e. 4-hourly) dose would require approximately 30 boosts. Each 'boost' advances the plunger only 0.23 mm delivering a completely inadequate dose of opioid analgesic and shortening the infusion time by about 8 min. Several extra 'boosts' thus not only significantly shorten the overall infusion time so that the CSCI finishes earlier than expected, but a higher dose of other drugs that might be in combination is delivered, which might be inappropriate.

16.3.2 **Changing from oral drugs to a CSCI**

If pain is controlled on an oral opioid, the CSCI can be commenced at the time the next oral dose is due, especially if it is a modified release preparation. If pain is not controlled, the CSCI should be started as soon as possible and a subcutaneous breakthrough (4-hourly) dose should be given as the CSCI is set up.

16.3.3 **Terminal phase**

In the terminal phase, usual current practice is to continue transdermal fentanyl or buprenorphine in patients stabilized on transdermal opioids. Any increase in pain can be managed with the addition of a CSCI of opioids via a syringe driver.

16.3.4 **Diluents**

The ideal diluent for CSCIs is still unclear. For most opioids, sterile water for injection, normal saline or 5% dextrose can all be used. Often, saline is preferred as it approximates to physiological tonicity, however, for concentrations of diamorphine greater than 40 mg/mL or opioid combinations containing cyclizine, where there is a risk of precipitating the chloride salt, then water for injection should be used.

16.3.5 **Infusion sites for CSCI**

Most infusions are delivered via a fine gauge butterfly needle or plastic cannula, inserted at 30–45° into the subcutaneous tissue. It is common practice to form a loop of tubing around this secured in place with a clear adhesive dressing to decrease the risk of the needle being dislodged. Usual infusion sites are the upper chest, anterior abdomen or thigh. The outer upper arm may be used, but is best avoided in cachectic patients where there is a high chance of displacement or discomfort. In confused or agitated patients, the inaccessible area over the scapula may be preferred. Areas of inflamed or broken skin, tumour infiltration, skin folds and oedematous or lymphoedematous areas should be avoided. Some infusion sites may remain intact for several days, particularly if single agent opioids are used. Conversely, with certain drugs or combinations, for example, cyclizine or methadone, site changes may be required daily.

16.3.6 **Problem solving**

Many opioids have a low pH in solution. Should inflammation at the infusion site persist, the following options should be considered:

- Decrease the concentration by increasing volume of diluent.
- Consider changing drivers every 12 h.
- Change infusion site regularly, for example, every 3 days or less.
- Change the drug combination or route.
- Change diluent to normal saline.
- Use non-metal cannula.
- Add hydrocortisone 50–100 mg or dexamethasone 0.5–1 mg (may be incompatible with some drugs).
- Inject hyaluronidase (enzyme said to break down connective tissue locally and aid diffusion) into site prior to starting CSCI.

16.4 **Opioids for CSCI**

16.4.1 **Weak opioids**

In the UK codeine, dihydrocodeine and tramadol are hardly ever used via CSCI, though in parts of the world where access to morphine is difficult, they may have a place. Parenterally, 120 mg of codeine, 60 mg of dihydrocodeine and 100 mg of tramadol are equivalent to 10 mg of parenteral morphine.

16.4.2 **Strong opioids**

16.4.2.1 *Morphine*

This remains the opioid of choice in managing cancer pain by mouth and became the parenteral opioid of choice in the UK during a national shortage of diamorphine. Dose escalation may be limited by volume when using Graseby syringe drivers.

Conversion ratio:	Oral morphine:parenteral morphine— 2:1–3:1 (DoH guidelines 2:1).
Initial starting dose:	Changing from step II opioids: 10–15 mg/24 h. Opioid-naïve patients and the elderly: 5–10 mg/24 h.
Cautions:	Metabolites are renally excreted so use with care in renal impairment.
Preparations:	10, 15, 20, 30 mg/mL, 1 and 2 mL ampoules.

16.4.2.2 *Diamorphine*

Diamorphine's significant advantage over morphine is its very high solubility; 1 g of diamorphine sulphate dissolves in 1.6 mL of water to give 2.4 mL in total (1 g of morphine sulphate requires 21 mL to dissolve). This leads to fewer problems of compatibility with other drugs and higher doses of the opioid can be given via CSCI. There is currently a national shortage of diamorphine in the UK.

Conversion ratio:	Oral morphine:parenteral diamorphine—3:1.
Initial starting dose:	Changing from step II opioids: 10 mg/24 h. Opioid-naïve patients and the elderly: 5–10 mg/24 h.
Cautions:	Metabolites are renally excreted so use with care in renal impairment.
Preparations:	5, 10, 30, 100, 500 mg ampoules.

16.4.2.3 *Oxycodone*

Oxycodone injection may be useful for patients already controlled on the oral preparation. Current concentrations available preclude high doses of opioid being delivered via syringe driver.

Conversion ratio:	Oral morphine: parenteral oxycodone—3:1. Oral oxycodone: parenteral oxycodone—2:1.
Initial starting dose:	Changing from step II opioids: 10 mg/24 h. Opioid-naïve patients and the elderly: 5–10 mg/24 h.
Cautions:	Despite inactive metabolites, plasma concentrations of oxycodone can accumulate in renal impairment.
Preparations:	10 mg/mL, 1 and 2 mL ampoules.

16.4.2.4 Hydromorphone

Hydromorphone is useful when diamorphine is not available, hence its widespread use in the USA and Australia. It is useful where small volumes of injection are needed.

Conversion ratio:	Oral morphine:parenteral hydromorphone 15:1. Oral hydromorphone:parenteral hydromorphone 2:1.
Initial starting dose:	2 mg/24 h.
Cautions:	Hydromorphone and its metabolites are renally excreted so use with care in renal impairment. In the UK it is used off licence on a named patient basis.
Preparations:	1, 2, 4 and 10 mg/mL in North America.

16.4.2.5 Fentanyl and its analogues

In palliative care fentanyl, sufentanil and alfentanil have all been used in CSCIs.

16.4.2.5.1 Fentanyl

Fentanyl can be used as a CSCI. Parenteral and transdermal fentanyl are equipotent.

Conversion ratio:	Oral morphine: parenteral fentanyl 100–150:1.
Initial starting dose:	Same as previous patch delivery over 24 h or 25 µg/h (with 12.5 µg boluses). Usual range is 500–4000 µg/h.
Cautions:	Difficult to deliver high doses via syringe driver because of large volumes. Fentanyl and its metabolites are not renally excreted so it is safe in renal failure.
Preparations:	As fentanyl citrate: 50 µg/mL, 2 and 10 mL ampoules.

16.4.2.5.2 Alfentanil

Alfentanil may be useful where small volumes of dilution are needed, therefore it is a suitable alternative to diamorphine especially in renal failure

Conversion ratio:	Oral morphine: parenteral alfentanil 30:1. Parenteral diamorphine:parenteral alfentanil 10:1. Approximately one-fourth potency of fentanyl.
Initial starting dose:	Opioid-naïve patients 0.5–1 mg/24 h.
Cautions:	Metabolized by CYP3A4 so dose may need to be reduced in hepatic impairment. Alfentanil and its metabolites are not renally excreted so it is safe in renal failure. May not mix with cyclizine; water for injection is required as the diluent.
Preparations:	500 µg/mL, 2 and 10 mL ampoules, 5 mg/mL, 1 mL ampoule.

16.4.2.5.3 Sufentanil

Sufentanil is usually used in anaesthesia. It may be useful for those patients previously on or needing fentanyl, when the volume required for CSCI is too great.

Conversion ratio: Parenteral fentanyl: parenteral sufentanil 7–10:1.
Cautions: Sufentanil is used in North America, Australia and New Zealand, and Europe but is not available in the UK.
Preparations: 50 µg/mL, 1, 2 and 5 mL ampoules.

16.4.2.6 *Buprenorphine*

The advent of the buprenorphine matrix patch should make its already rare use via a CSCI obsolete.

16.4.2.7 *Methadone*

Methadone is difficult to use because of its long and variable half-life. Its use via a CSCI should be limited usually to those patients previously stabilized on oral methadone who are no longer able to take oral drugs.

Conversion ratio: Oral methadone:parenteral methadone 2:1.
Cautions: Long half-life, so can accumulate. Irritation at infusion site may be a problem. Avoid concurrent cimetidine, fluoxetine and monoamine oxidase inhibitors. Methadone and its metabolites are not renally excreted so safe for use in renal impairment.
Preparations: 10 mg/mL, 1, 2, 3.5 and 5 mL ampoules.

16.5 **Stability and compatibility**

There are several excellent and detailed charts and tables, particularly Dickman *et al.* (2005) and Twycross *et al.* (2002) giving the stability and physical and chemical compatibility of the various drugs used commonly in CSCIs. Factors which may cause problems with compatibility include the number of different drugs used in combination, their concentration and the diluent used.

16.6 **Intravenous opioids**

The intravenous route is not generally favoured for the delivery of opioids in palliative care, unless the patient is in a postoperative setting or, rarely, has particular reasons for requiring patient controlled analgesia, however, it has its protagonists. At Memorial Sloan-Kettering Cancer Centre a commonly employed strategy is to titrate patients to pain control using IV methadone where pain is not responding to other opioids.

Where severe pain calls for rapid titration, Harris and colleagues (2003) describe a regimen using IV boluses of 1.5 mg morphine given every 10 min until the patient develops drowsiness or achieves pain control (80%). Thereafter, 4-hourly oral morphine can be given at a dose equivalent to the total IV dose; 95% of patients need less than 15 mg. The same dose is then used for breakthrough pain.

The advantages of this IV regimen are

- Rapid pain relief.
- Ability to estimate quickly the patient's opioid requirements.
- Ability to determine quickly whether the pain is responsive to opioids.

On the basis that morphine's hydrophilicity can delay its peak effect, IV fentanyl has been advocated for use in 'fast titration' during cancer pain emergencies. Using a breakthrough dose of one-fifth of the equivalent oral daily dose of morphine, Mercadante and colleagues (2004) report IV fentanyl to be safe and effective in the majority of patients. The same group also describe its use for breakthrough pain in patients whose background analgesia is transdermal buprenorphine. Such regimens should, however, be used with caution since repeated boluses of morphine and diamorphine IV can lead to tachyphylaxis, that is, acute tolerance to the analgesic effect.

16.7 **Conclusion**

Although different opioid formulations and routes of administration are increasingly available, when the oral route is not suitable, the mainstay of good analgesia in cancer related pain remains the use of strong opioids via a CSCI. Because of its high solubility, diamorphine is the preferred opioid in the UK and was the most frequently used until it became scarce. The choice of alternative opioid for CSCI, including morphine, oxycodone, hydromorphone and alfentanil, will depend upon the patient's current opioid, the dose needed and whether the volume of drug will be limited by the infusion device to be used.

Key references

Anderson, R., Soiers, J.H., Abrams, S. and Schlicht, C. (2001). Accuracy in equianalgesic dosing: Conversion dilemmas. *J. Pain Symptom Manage.*, **21**, 397–406.

Dickman, A., Schneider, J. and Varga, J. (2005). *The syringe driver*, 2nd edn. Oxford University Press, Oxford.

Hanks, G.W., Conno, F., Cherny, N., Hanna, M., Kalso, E., *et al.* (2001). Morphine and alternative opioids in cancer pain: The EAPC recommendations. *Br. J. Cancer.*, **84**, 587–93.

Harris, J.T., Kumar, K.S. and Rajagopal, M.R. (2003). Intravenous morphine for rapid control of severe cancer pain. *Palliat. Med.*, **17**, 248–56.

Herndon, C.M. and Fike, D.S. (2001). Continuous subcutaneous infusion practices of USA Hospices. *J. Pain Symptom Manage.*, **22,** 1027–34.

Manfredi, P.L., Foley, K.M., Payne, R., Houde, R. and Inturrisi, C.E. (2003). Parenteral methadone: an essential medication for the treatment of pain. *J. Pain Symptom Manage.*, **26**, 687–8.

Mercadante, S., Villari, P., Ferrera, P., Bianchi, M. and Casuccio, A. (2004). Safety and effectiveness of intravenous morphine for episodic breakthrough pain using a fixed ratio with the oral daily morphine dose. *J. Pain Symptom Manage.*, **27**, 352–9.

Mercadante, S., Villari, P., Ferrera, P., Porzio, G., Aielli, F. and Verna, L. (2006). Safety and effectiveness of intravenous morphine for episodic breakthrough pain in patients receiving transdermal buprenorphine. *J. Pain Symptom Manage.*, **32**, 175–9.

Murray, A. and Hagen, N.A. (2005). Hydromorphone. *J. Pain Symptom Manage.*, **29**, (S5), 57–66.

Negro, S., Martin, A., Azuara, M., Sanchez, Y. and Barcia, E. (2005). Stability of tramadol and haloperidol for continuous subcutaneous infusion at home. *J. Pain Symptom Manage.*, **30**, 192–9.

Pereira, J., Lawlor, P., Vigaro, A., Dogan, M. and Bruera, E. (2001). Equianalgesic dose ratios for opioids: critical review and proposals for long term dosing. *J. Pain Symptom Manage.*, **22**, 672–87.

Soares, L.G., Martins, M. and Uchoa, R. (2003). Intravenous fentanyl for cancer pain: a "fast titration" protocol for the emergency room. *J. Pain Symptom Manage.*, **26**, 876–81.

Takahashi, M., Ohara, T., Yamanaka, H., Shimada, A., Nakaho, T. and Yamamuro, M. (2003). The oral-to-intravenous equianalgesic ratio of morphine based on plasma concentrations of morphine and metabolites in advanced cancer patients receiving chronic morphine treatment. *Palliat. Med.*, **17**, 673–8.

Twycross, R., Wilcock, A., Charlesworth, S. and Dickman, A. (2002). *Palliative care formulary*, 2nd edn. Radcliffe Medical Press, Oxford.

Wilcock, A., Jacob, J.K., Charlesworth, S., Harris, E., Gibbs, M. and Allsop, H. (2006). Drugs given by a syringe driver: a prospective multicentre survey of palliative care services in the UK. *Palliat. Med.*, **7**, 661–4.

Chapter 17

Opioids in special circumstances

Fliss Murtagh, Polly Edmonds and Chris Farnham

Key points

Opioids in renal disease:

- The degree of renal impairment should be established where possible, using estimated glomerular filtration rate.
- Choice of opioid is important.
- In severe renal impairment, avoid repeated administration of opioids with known toxic metabolites (such as codeine, dihydrocodeine, morphine and diamorphine), and avoid modified release preparations.
- Use preferred opioids (buprenorphine, fentanyl and alfentanil) carefully, start at very low doses, with increased dose interval, and titrate against clinical response.

Opioids in liver disease:

- Many patients with hepatic dysfunction have pain requiring opioid analgesics.
- The liver dysfunction needs to be severe for clinical issues around prescribing in palliative care to become relevant.
- Avoid opioids with long half lives and modified release preparations; if toxicity develops, it will be prolonged.
- Opioids should be used with caution eg low starting doses, increased dose interval and careful monitoring.
- Alternative opioids do not have any specific advantages.

Opioids in respiratory disease:

- Opioids are known to have respiratory depressant side effects.
- Clinicians may be anxious about prescribing opioids in patients with chronic lung disease.

Key points (*Contd.*)

- In practice, patients seem to develop tolerance to the respiratory depressant side effects.
- Careful titration with normal release opioids and regular clinical review means these drugs can be used in patients with respiratory disease.

Prescribing opioids in patients with a history of drug misuse:

- Patients with a history of substance misuse develop pain.
- Substance misuse can be a barrier to adequate pain management.
- Effective pain control requires good communication, boundary setting and team working.
- British Pain Society guidance should guide practice.

17.1 **Opioids in renal disease**

17.1.1 **Opioid metabolism**

The majority of opioids are metabolized in the liver, and the parent drug and its metabolites are mostly excreted via the kidney, with some important exceptions. Because of this, the main risk of opioid use in renal impairment is rapid accumulation of metabolites and/or the parent drug, and subsequent toxicity because of this accumulation. The analgesic and adverse effects of opioid metabolites are variable; for this reason, the effect of renal failure on individual opioids varies considerably. The most important considerations when using any individual opioid are

- What is the level of renal impairment, since this will most affect accumulation of parent drug and metabolites if they are excreted mainly through the kidney?
- Are there other routes of excretion?
- What effects do the metabolites have, especially as they accumulate?
- What effects does the parent drug have, especially as it accumulates?
- Is the patient receiving dialysis or not?

17.1.2 **The level of renal impairment**

It is important to calculate the estimated glomerular filtration rate (eGFR) and not to rely on serum creatinine alone because eGFR is a much more accurate reflection of renal function. Much of the discussion in this section relates to Stage 5 chronic kidney disease (eGFR <15 mL/min), but it applies to a lesser extent in Stages 3 and 4 too (Table 17.1).

17.1.3 Using opioids in renal disease

Barakzoy and Moss (2006) have evaluated the World Health Organization (WHO) analgesic ladder in patients with renal insufficiency and suggest that it leads to effective treatment of pain in >90% of haemodialysis patients. Table 17.2 summarizes the main considerations and recommendations for practice when patients are not on dialysis. If a patient is on regular dialysis, it is also important to consider whether an opioid is removed during dialysis; those opioids with high molecular weight, low water solubility, and high protein binding and volume of distribution (such as fentanyl, alfentanil and methadone), are unlikely to be removed by dialysis. Drugs with relatively low protein binding and moderate solubility, such as morphine and diamorphine, may be removed by dialysis.

Table 17.1 Stages of chronic kidney disease	
Chronic kidney disease	eGFR
Stage 3	30–59 mL/min
Stage 4	15–29 mL/min
Stage 5	<15 mL/min

17.1.4 Summary—opioids in renal disease

Ideally, drugs with a short half-life should be used. If accumulation occurs, it is easier to discontinue them quickly. Modified release or long-acting preparations should be avoided. Doses should be reduced and the dose interval increased. The patient should be monitored frequently, especially when the opioid is first commenced since accumulation and adverse effects can occur within a few hours of a single dose and late accumulation may also occur despite a stable opioid regimen.

17.2 Opioids in liver disease

17.2.1 Opioid absorption

Most opioids have good oral absorption. Theoretically the presence of ascites may reduce absorption; this may be more significant for drugs which are incompletely or variably absorbed, for example, morphine or hydromorphone.

17.2.2 Distribution

The more water soluble opioids will distribute into ascites, resulting in a reduction in concentration of circulating drug. In cachectic patients with less fat, higher concentrations of more lipid soluble opioids (e.g. alfentanil, fentanyl) may occur and both low albumin and a high bilirubin can increase the free fraction and hence activity of highly protein bound drugs (e.g. fentanyl and methadone).

17.2.3 **Metabolism**

The metabolism of opioids appears to be well preserved during periods of acute liver dysfunction, but can become altered in advanced disease.

The pharmacokinetics of opioids may be influenced by

- Hepatic blood flow (reduced clearance of metabolites).
- Cirrhosis.
- Cardiac failure.
- Porto-systemic shunts.
- Enzyme capacity of liver ($\uparrow$ PT or INR suggests severe dysfunction).
- Type of drug metabolism (oxidation/glucuronidation).
- Protein binding.
- Cholestasis.

17.2.4 **Using opioids in liver disease**

The key principles of using opioids in liver disease are as follows

- Ideally use drugs with a short half-life.
- If PT/INR raised or albumin decreased consider dose reduction.
- Start with a small dose and increase slowly or use 'as required' dosing. Monitor patient closely.

Note that all opioid analgesics can precipitate hepatic encephalopathy, due to altered pharmacokinetics, increased receptor sensitivity and their tendency to cause constipation (Table 17.3).

17.3 **Opioids in respiratory disease**

17.3.1 **Background**

Clinicians may be concerned when prescribing opioids for pain in patients with end-stage respiratory disease in view of the potential respiratory depressant effects of all opioid analgesics. This is particularly so where there is type II respiratory failure (low oxygen levels associated with a high carbon dioxide), where it is feared opioids might precipitate or exacerbate respiratory failure.

However, although it is well recognized that opioids can cause respiratory depression, in clinical practice this is rarely relevant as patients appear to develop tolerance to the respiratory depressant effects with repeated dosing.

Table 17.2 Recommendations for opioid use in renal disease without dialysis

WHO analgesic ladder	Opioid	Metabolites	Excretion	Toxicity	Recommendations at each stage of chronic kidney disease
Step 2	Codeine and Dihydrocodeine	Many active metabolites (norcodeine, codeine-6-glucuronide, morphine, normorphine, morphine-3-glucuronide and morphine-6-glucuronide)	Predominantly renal	Risk of severe hypotension, respiratory depression and arrest, sedation and profound narcolepsy.	Reduce dose and increase dose interval in Stage 3 and 4. Not recommended in Stage 5.
Step 2	Tramadol	Only one active metabolite (O-demethyl-tramadol)	Predominantly renal	Usual opioids side effects, especially confusion and hallucinations. Epileptogenic as is uraemia itself).	Reduce dose and increase dose interval in Stage 3 and 4. Can be used in Stage 5, but maximum 50 mg every 12 h orally.
Step 3	Buprenorphine	Two main metabolites (norbuprenorphine and buprenorphine-3-glucuronide)	Metabolites are excreted renally, but buprenorphine is excreted mainly via the biliary system	Metabolites do accumulate in renal failure, but little evidence as yet to support or refute toxicity.	Theoretical reasons why it may be better than some other opioids but use with caution and reduce doses at all stages.

Table 17.2 (Contd.)

WHO analgesic ladder	Opioid	Metabolites	Excretion	Toxicity	Recommendations at each stage of chronic kidney disease
Step 3	Fentanyl and alfentanil	Metabolites largely inactive (norfentanyl and others)	Predominantly renal	Metabolites largely inactive and non-toxic. Parent drug may accumulate with sustained administration—note wide interpatient variability.	Preferred opioids in renal impairment; use constrained by limited formulations and availability. Opioid of choice for subcutaneous administration towards the end of life (Note: alfentanil has a short half-life and is best used only for continuous subcutaneous infusion).
Step 3	Hydromorphone	Active main metabolite (hydromorphone-3-glucuronide)	Predominantly renal	Hydromorphone-3-glucuronide accumulates in renal failure—it may be neuro excitatory but little evidence as yet.	In Stages 3 and 4, reduce dose and increase dose interval. In Stage 5, there is too little evidence to recommend use, although likely less risk of toxicity than with morphine/diamorphine.
Step 3	Methadone	Main metabolite 1,5-dimethyl-2-ethyl-3,3-diphenyl-1-pyrroline	Main metabolite is excreted f aecally, although unchanged drug is also excreted renally	Probably little accumulation in renal failure, and little added risk of toxicity.	Challenging to use, not because of the effects of renal failure, but because of wide interindividual variation, considerable difference between acute and chronic phase dosing, and accumulation of methadone on repeated administration due to its high volume of distribution. Use as normal in

Step 3					Stages 3 and 4 (reduce dose by 50% in Stage 5). (Experienced specialist supervision of regime recommended at all stages.)
Step 3	Morphine and diamorphine	Several active metabolites (normorphine, morphine-3-glucuronide, and morphine-6-glucuronide)	Predominantly renal	Morphine-3-glucuronide has prolonged central nervous system (CNS) depressant effects. Morphine-3-glucuronide may antagonise analgesic effects and be neurotoxic.	In Stage 3 and 4, reduce dose and increase dose interval. Modified-release preparations should only be used very cautiously. In Stage 5, not recommended for use.
Step 3	Oxycodone	Active metabolites (noroxycodone, oxymorphone)	Predominantly renal	Very limited evidence; central nervous system toxicity and sedation have been reported.	In Stages 3 and 4, reduce dose and increase dose interval. In Stage 5, there is too little evidence to recommend use, although likely less risk of toxicity than with morphine/diamorphine.

Table 17.3 Recommendations for opioid use in liver disease

Drug	Key points
Opioids for mild to moderate pain	
Tramadol	• Opioid effects reduced due to altered liver metabolism but serotonin/noradrenalin properties expected to increase—overall effect not clear • Altered pharmacokinetics—increase dosing interval in renal and hepatic disease • Increased sensitivity—encephalopathy • Constipation—encephalopathy
Codeine/dihydrocodeine	• Scarcity of information available • Codeine relies on metabolism to be converted to active morphine so patients with chronic liver disease MAY derive less analgesia from codeine • Not recommended
Opioids for moderate to severe pain	
Morphine	• High hepatic extraction ratio and large first pass metabolism • Hepatic impairment may increase systemic availability • Studies suggest that metabolism of morphine is significantly impaired in patients with severe cirrhosis • Recommendations: 　• Reduce oral doses ± increase dosing interval 　• Increased systemic availability less of an issue with SC dosing BUT caution required
Oxycodone	• End-stage cirrhosis reduces the clearance and increases the half-life of oxycodone • Recommendations: 　• Dose reduction may be required in advanced disease
Methadone	• Normal doses of methadone may be used in mild to moderate liver impairment • Methadone likely to accumulate in severe liver disease • Recommendations: 　• Careful monitoring and dose reductions likely to be required in severe liver disease

Drug	Key points
Fentanyl	• Limited information but appears as if fentanyl pharmacokinetics are relatively unaffected by hepatocyte dysfunction BUT may be affected by severe liver dysfunction or reduced hepatic blood flow • Recommendations: • Careful monitoring, particularly for CNS effects, and consider dose reduction in severe disease
Alfentanil	• Half-life, clearance and protein binding of alfentanil all shown to be reduced in cirrhotic patients • Effect of alfentanil may be enhanced and prolonged • Recommendations: • Use with caution in those with liver impairment

Table 17.3 (Contd.)

17.3.2 Evidence of tolerability

Walsh studied 20 patients with advanced cancer requiring strong opioid analgesia, 12 of these patients had a history of chronic lung disease. Twelve patients were hypoxic but only one had a raised pCO_2 suggesting that respiratory failure was uncommon in this patient group. This finding has been supported by a recent study demonstrating that opioid titration is not associated with significant respiratory depression and by Jennings' systematic review of the use of opioids for managing breathlessness of any cause, where there was no evidence that the use of opioids was associated with adverse effects on arterial blood gases or oxygen saturation in the populations studied.

17.3.3 Clinical practice

In practice, careful titration of opioid analgesics with regular clinical review, initially with normal release preparations, should enable safe and effective use of opioids, by allowing tolerance to develop to the respiratory depressant effect of morphine.

17.4 Prescribing opioids in patients with a history of drug misuse

17.4.1 The problem of drug misuse

The proportion of the population of the USA estimated to have a substance use disorder varies between 6% and 15%. In chronic pain services in the USA some studies suggest up to 41% of patients receiving chronic pain management are abusing opioids. In the UK, this proportion among palliative care patients is unknown, but is thought to be small. Whilst the British Pain Society issued guidance in 2006, this does not cover all of the issues surrounding a palliative care patient with misuse issues.

Up to 90% patients who are dying with metastatic cancer experience some pain and this figure can rise if the patient has a history of substance misuse. A small study at Memorial Sloan-Kettering Cancer Center showed that 3% of all consultations to the psychiatry service were about substance misuse. This almost certainly under-represents the true incidence of a problem which is missed because of poor access to palliative care and other tertiary services, to health professionals' ignorance about how to identify such patients and to patients' and professionals' fears about stigmatisation.

17.4.2 Terminology

- Addiction is a syndrome and pattern of substance misuse and describes continued drug use despite harm.
- Dependence on a substance describes the state of requiring the substance to prevent physiological withdrawal, which can occur in addiction or in a non-addicted patient.
- Pseudo-addiction is the seeking of drugs, often associated with aberrant behaviour, due primarily to poor analgesic control.

17.4.3 Why do people become addicted?

Mu receptor stimulation leads to the release of dopamine in the meso-cortico-limbic system and leads to a suppression of noradrenaline in the locus coeruleus. This explains the feeling of well-being and also the feelings of 'cold turkey' on withdrawal, secondary to the surge of noradrenalin released.

17.4.4 Patient group

It is important to recognize that patients with substance misuse disorder may develop pain due to malignancy. They also often have multiple medical comorbidities, such as mental health problems, cardiovascular disease, respiratory problems and poor nutrition that may cause or exacerbate pain. They are often socially disadvantaged and have a higher incidence of family members who misuse drugs.

17.4.5 Barriers

Patients who are actively misusing drugs and alcohol present some of the most challenging pain management problems. They have the greatest risk of diversion of drugs and often the pain becomes a barrier to treatment of their addiction.

17.4.5.1 *Management plan*

- Assess the misuse history at an early stage. By being clear and open, the team is able to take a non-judgemental position. Careful documentation is needed to prevent prejudicial treatment from other professionals (Table 17.4).
- Use the multidisciplinary team, including pharmacist, mental health worker, palliative care team, substance misuse team and chronic pain team. Involve primary care—it is where the patient will be spending most of their time.
- Identify any pre-existing mental health problems and evaluate and treat.
- Set goals that are realistic for the patient. Of the patients with addiction problems, 80% will relapse within 1 year. Total compliance and abstinence might not be achievable. Frequent team meetings for goal readjustment might be needed.
- Treat the pain properly. Individualization of the drug dose needed to achieve analgesia is important and tolerance might necessitate large doses. Prescribers who are unsure of opioid use might find these large doses difficult to prescribe leading to withholding or assumptions about aberrant behaviour. Withholding correct doses can in turn lead to withdrawal or pseudo-addictive behaviour.

17.4.5.2 *Contracts*

The relationship between patient and prescriber relies on trust and with that trust must come an explicit set of rules. The two parties agreeing to rules that define clearly the consequences of aberrant behaviour can set boundaries for care. These rules have to be structured for individuals and the clinical setting. Kirsh suggests clear agreement about what happens with prescription loss or adjustment and suggests that there should be only one named prescriber with covering clinicians being made aware of the contract.

Table 17.4 Brief summary of British Pain Society guidance for substance misusers
Choose long-acting or modified release opioids where possible
Limit or eliminate normal release and short-acting breakthrough analgesics
Maximize the use of non-opioid adjuvants
Maximize the use of non-drug treatments (transcutaneous electrical nerve stimulation (TENS), Cognitive Behavioural Therapy)
Think about limiting the total dose dispensed at any one time
Use pill count and urine screens as necessary
Use the local substance misuse team

Table 17.5 Examples of drug interactions and their effects

Misused drug	Prescribed drugs and effect of interaction
All	Care with HIV antiretrovirals
All	Anti-TB medication
Opioids	Alcohol potentiates CNS effects
Opioids	Benzodiazepines potentiate CNS effects
Opioids	Cannabis potentiates CNS effects
Methadone/buprenorphine	Carbamazepine—increased opioid metabolism-possible withdrawal effects
Methadone/buprenorphine	Phenytoin—increased opioid metabolism-possible withdrawal effects
Methadone	Tricyclics—theoretical additive effect on prolongation QT interval leading to arrhythmias
Opioids	Tricyclics—potentiated CNS effects

17.4.5.3 *Drug interactions*

Clinicians need to be aware of the possibility of drug interactions between both prescribed and misused drugs. Examples are given in Table 17.5.

17.4.6 **Summary**

Patients with a history of substance abuse develop pain due to malignancy and/or other comorbidities. There is a real danger their pain will be inadequately managed. British Pain Society guidance is helpful and includes using modified release preparations where possible in association with adjuvant drugs and non-drug measures. Successful pain management requires open communication, clear boundary and goal setting and multidisciplinary team input.

Key references

Barakzoy, A.S. and Moss, A.H. (2006). Efficacy of the world health organization analgesic ladder to treat pain in end-stage renal disease. *J. Am. Soc. Nephrol.*, **17**, 3198–203.

British Pain Society (2006). *Pain and substance misuse: improving the patient experience. Consensus document.* British Pain Society, London.

Dean, M. (2004). Opioids in renal failure and dialysis patients. *J. Pain Symptom Manage.*, **28**, 497–504.

Estfan, B., Mahmoud, F., Shaheen, P., Davis, M.P., Lasheen, W., Rivera, N., et al. (2007). Respiratory function during parenteral opioid titration for cancer pain. *Palliat. Med.*, **21**, 81–6.

Gonzales, G.R. (1992). Treatment of cancer pain in a former opioid abuser: fears of the patient and staff and their influences on care. *J. Pain Symptom Manage.*, **7**, 246–9.

Jennings, A.L., Davies, A.N., Higgins, J.P., Gibbs, J.S. and Broadley, K.E. (2002). A systematic review of the use of opioids in the management of dyspnoea. *Thorax*, **57**, 939–44.

Kemp, C. (1996). Managing chronic pain in patients with advanced disease and substance related disorders. *Home Healthc. Nurse*, **14**, 225–61.

Kirsh, K.L. (2006). Palliative care of the terminally ill drug addict. *Cancer Invest.*, **24**, 425–31.

Manchikanti, L. (2006). Controlled substance abuse and illicit drug use in chronic pain patients: an evaluation of multiple variables. *Pain Physician*, **9**, 215–25.

Murtagh, F.E.M., Chai, M.O., Donohoe, P., Edmonds, P.M. and Higginson, I.J. (2007). The use of opioid analgesia in end-stage renal disease patients managed without dialysis. recommendations for practice. *J. Pain Palliat. Care Pharmacother.* (in press).

Passik, S.D. (1998). Substance abuse issues in cancer patients. Part 2: evaluation and treatment. *Oncology (Williston Park)*, **12**, 729–34.

Scalc, J.P. and Muramoto, M.L. (1993). Substance abuse among minority populations. *Prim. Care*, **20**, 167–80.

Volles, D.F. and McGory, R. (1999). Perspectives in pain management—pharmacokinetic considerations. *Crit. Care Clin.*, **15**, 55–75.

Walsh, T.D. (1984). Opiates and respiratory function in advanced cancer. *Recent Results Cancer Res.*, **89**, 115–7.

Dose conversion when switching from oral morphine to transdermal fentanyl

Dose conversion		
4-hourly morphine (mg) (also breakthrough medication dose)	Fentanyl patch strength (µg/h)	24-hourly oral morphine dose (mg)
<20*	25	<90
20*	37	90 to 134
25 to 30*	50	135 to 189
35*	62	190 to 224
40 to 50	75	225 to 314
55 to 65	100	315 to 404
70 to 80	125	405 to 494
85 to 95	150	495 to 584
100 to 110	175	585 to 674
110 to 125	200	675 to 764
130 to 140	225	765 to 854
145 to 155	250	855 to 944
160 to 170	275	945 to 1034
175 to 185	300	1035 to 1124

* 4-hourly morphine doses <40–50 mg calculated by editor. These are <u>NOT</u> supplied in the Summary of Product Characteristics for Durogesic DTrans®.

Adapted from Summary of Product Characteristics for Durogesic DTrans®, Janssen-Cilag Ltd.

Index

Please note that references to non-textual material such as Figures or Tables are in *italic* print